The Safety Book for Active Kids

Teaching Your Child How to Avoid Everyday Dangers

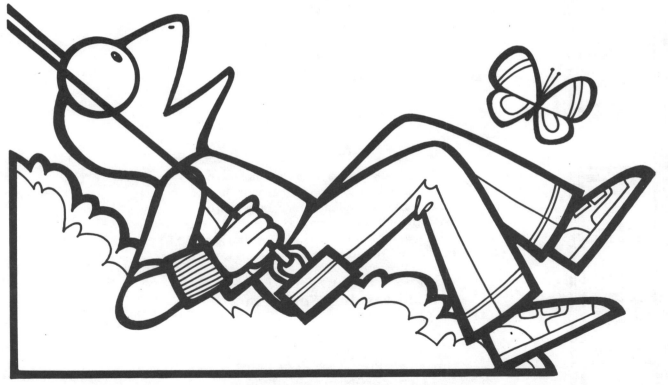

Written by Linda Schwartz • Illustrated by Bev Armstrong

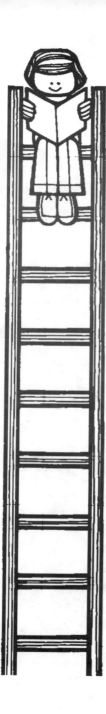

The Learning Works

Cover Design & Illustration:
Beverly Armstrong

Text Design and Editorial Production:
Kimberley A. Clark

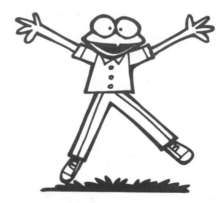

Copyright © 1995—Linda Schwartz

The Learning Works, Inc.

P.O. Box 6187
Santa Barbara, California 93160

ISBN: 0-88160-270-1
Library of Congress: 95-079752

Dedication

This book is dedicated with love
to my parents,
Ina and William Schwartz.

❧

Thanks for keeping me safe
through hurricanes, mishaps, and
all the perils of growing up.

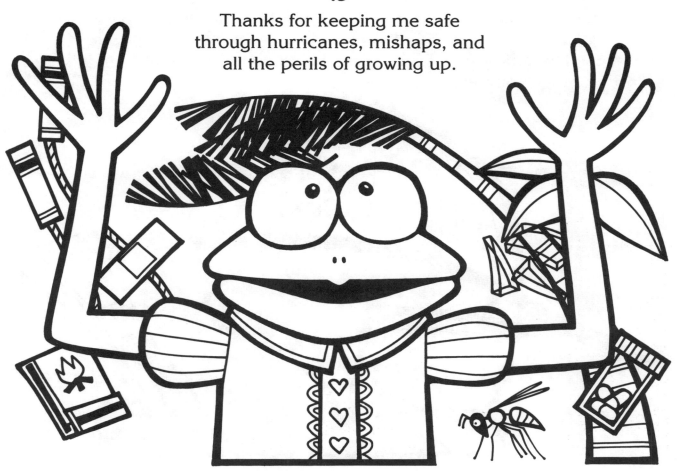

Acknowledgments

Special thanks to Officer Tom Regalie of the Santa Barbara Police Department; to Diane Lantz, Director of Health and Safety at the Santa Barbara chapter of the American Red Cross; and to Captain Charlie Johnson and Katherine Lynn of the Santa Barbara County Fire Department.

Thanks also go to Dr. Stephen Abbott and Bobbie Vidal, LMFCC, for their comments and suggestions.

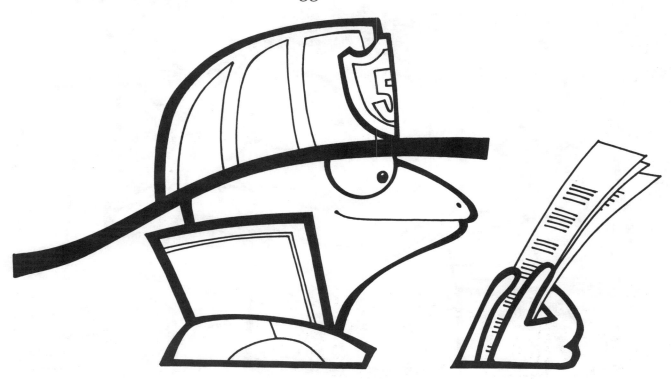

Contents

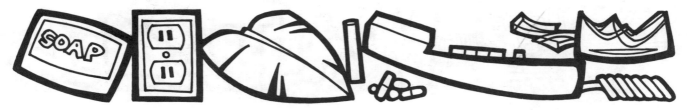

Contents
(continued)

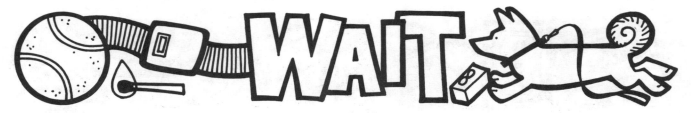

Contents
(continued)

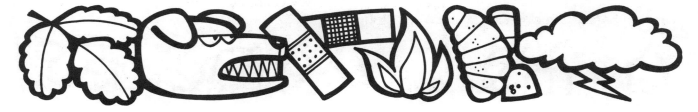

7

Contents
(continued)

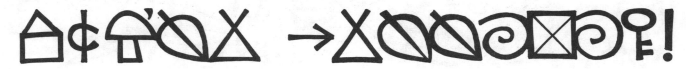

A Note to Kids

Have you ever been lost or frightened? Have you injured yourself when you were alone? Found something dangerous? Worried about thunderstorms, accidents, or fires?

Part of growing up is finding out about things that can happen to you—things that are confusing, scary, or dangerous. Another part of growing up is learning what you can do to keep yourself, your family, and your friends safe.

When you read *The Safety Book for Active Kids* with your mom, dad, or another adult, you will be able to talk about some of the things that can happen. Together, you and your mom or dad can decide what to do and how to stay safe. You can make plans for things that might happen at home, at school, at play, or out and about. Planning ahead of time makes doing the safe thing much easier.

Sit down with your mom or dad and pick a page that looks interesting. Read the situation. Think about what you might do. Come up with as many ideas as you can. Then turn the page and have mom or dad read the steps that are suggested. Talk about them with your parents and decide what you would do if you were ever in that situation.

Dangerous or scary situations don't seem as bad when you already know what to do. You can practice safety just like you practice reading or swimming. If you make a safety plan and practice what to do, you'll know how to keep yourself and others safe.

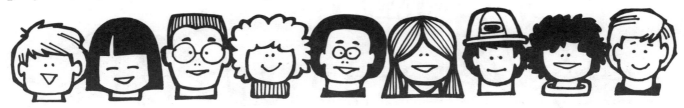

A Note to Parents

A stray dog, a loaded gun, a house on fire, a stranger offering your child a ride—life is full of dangers for kids whether they are at home, at school, at play, or just out and about. How can you, as a concerned parent, help prepare your children for the world around them?

The Safety Book for Active Kids is filled with situations that children ages 4–8 might encounter. It is designed to help a child think about and plan for these situations beforehand so that he or she will be better prepared to deal with them if and when they arise. While most of the situations concern a child's physical safety, several deal with important issues such as homesickness and bed-wetting, which can affect a child's emotional well-being.

This is a book to read and share with your child. Of course, no one book can be all things to all children because no one can imagine all possible safety situations, anticipate all probable reactions, and/or describe all practical solutions. For these reasons, *The Safety Book for Active Kids* is intended to be used as a guide, not as a manual. It suggests a direction for your child to take, but it does not prescribe all of the steps that should be followed in getting there.

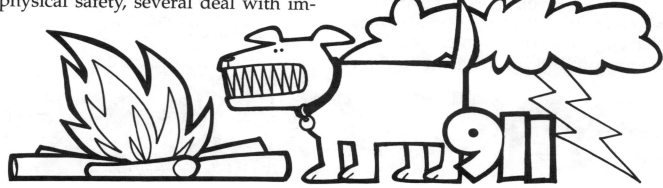

A Note to Parents
(continued)

As you read this book with your child, think about what actions are best for *your* family. Use the book to plan behaviors that are right and safe for your child and your situation.

Encourage your child to choose one of the situations in *The Safety Book for Active Kids*. Read it aloud and talk about the situation. Before you turn the page, ask your child what he or she would do in this situation. Help your child put his or her actions in order so that the most important things are done first.

Then have your child turn the page and compare his or her ideas with the steps listed. Talk about the similarities and differences and the reasons for them. Modify the steps that are listed to make them fit your specific family situation and the maturity and ability of your child.

The situations described in this book are ideal for dinner table discussions, for use while traveling, and for all those times you want to open the doors of communication with your child. They make the perfect springboard to discussions and help prepare your child for those times when he or she may face the unexpected.

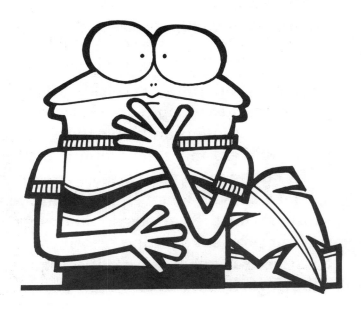

A Note to Teachers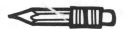

For a great way to begin each school morning, select a different topic for discussion each day. You could also develop an entire unit around a safety theme.

Fire Prevention Week

Use the pages on house fires in class and, for homework, have students take home copies of page 189 so they can plan and practice using fire escape routes with their families. Visit a local fire station to learn about fire hazards and then conduct a fire safety inspection of the classroom.

Bicycle Safety Week

Invite a police officer to visit the classroom and talk about bike safety and proper equipment. Read page 193 on selecting a bike helmet to your class, or have students work with the pages on riding double or losing a helmet. Have your students make a list of bicycle safety tips.

Home Safety

Photocopy several safety checklists for your students and let each family work together to make sure that home is a safe place. The situations in the "At Home" section will also help students recognize a number of home safety issues.

In addition, the situations in *The Safety Book for Active Kids* can be used for role playing and for cooperative learning. For example, you can assign parts to small groups of students and have them create simple skits by writing dialogue, finding props, and planning the action to demonstrate good safety practices.

By taking the time to discuss these situations with your students throughout the school year, you'll be helping them prepare for the unexpected. As they consider solutions for the various situations in the book, they will be developing skills in solving problems, setting priorities, and evaluating outcomes. The exercises can thus serve as vehicles for critical thinking and planning—and for promoting safe behavior with children.

At Home

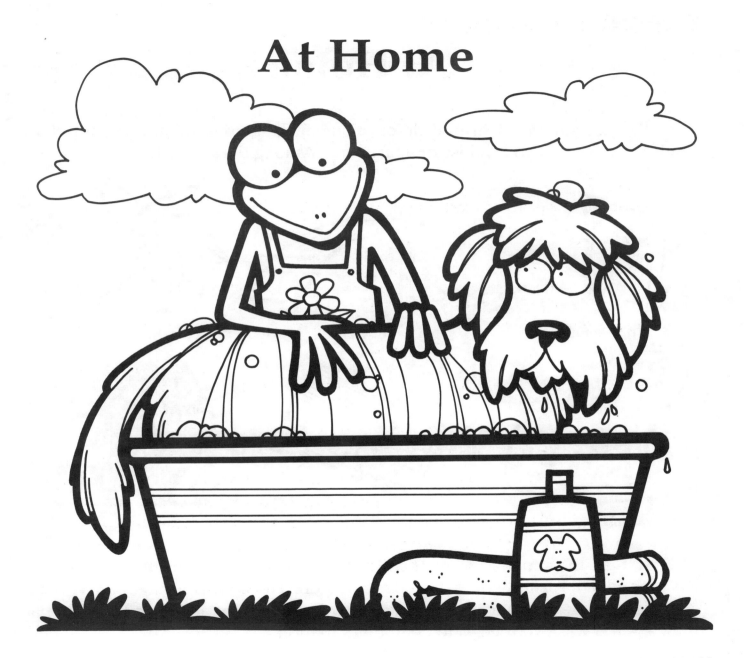

At Home

In this section, you will find descriptions of dangerous situations your child might encounter in your house or apartment. Among these situations are

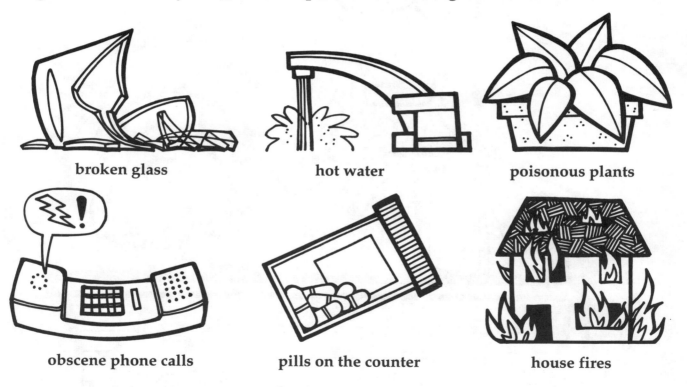

broken glass   hot water   poisonous plants

obscene phone calls   pills on the counter   house fires

First, read the situation to your child. Next, have your child think about and describe what he or she would do in this situation. Then, turn the page and read the steps listed there to your child. Finally, talk over these steps and discuss additional things you'd want your child to do in this situation.

Hot Water

You have been playing outside all morning,
and now your hands are covered with dirt.
You go to the kitchen sink to wash them.
You turn on the water, and you see steam rising
from the water that's coming out of the faucet.

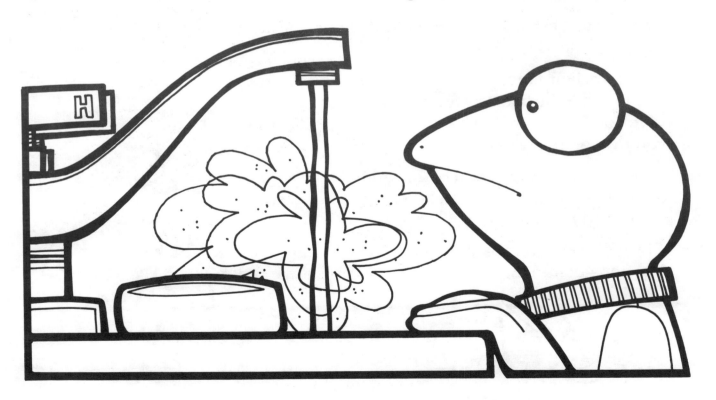

Hot Water

- Don't put your hands in the water. When water steams, it is too hot to touch. It can cause a serious and painful burn.

- Turn off the water. Then turn the cold water on first. Let it run to be sure it is cold. Then add hot water, a little at a time, until the water is warm.

- Often water gets hotter as it runs, so remember to add hot water slowly.

- Many kitchen faucets have only one handle. You push the handle one way for hot water and the other for cold. Make sure the handle is set for cold before you turn on the water.

- When you run water for a bath, add hot water carefully. Keep checking to make sure it's not getting hotter and hotter.

- Always check your bath water with your hand before you get into the tub.

Parents' Corner

In only **three seconds** a child can sustain a third-degree burn from water at 140° F. Such a severe burn can require hospitalization and skin grafts.

Be safe. Set the thermostat on your hot water heater no higher than 115° F.

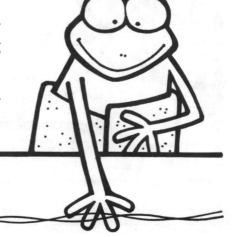

Electrical Outlets

One morning while you are watching television,
you see your baby sister crawl toward
an electrical outlet. She has your mother's keys,
and she pokes one of the keys at the outlet.

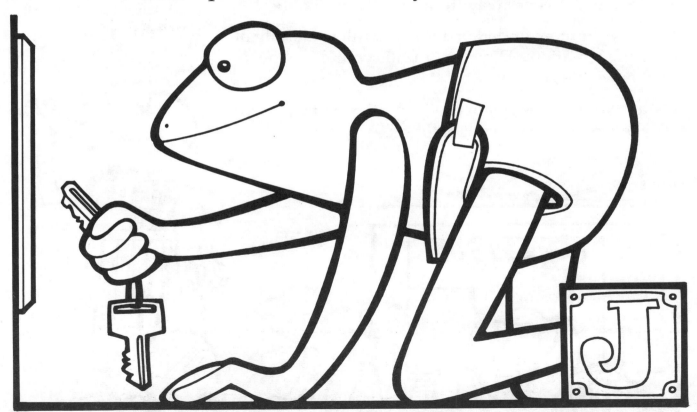

Electrical Outlets

- Quickly take away the keys—or any other object that a small child could poke into an outlet. Putting things into electrical outlets can cause shock or injury.

- Move your sister away from the electrical outlet.

- Call your mom or dad or another adult to alert them to the situation. Don't wait until your TV show is over.

- Take your baby sister or brother with you if you have to leave the room to get help.

Parents' Corner

Most hardware stores sell safety covers to fit over electrical outlets. To keep small children safe in your home, put safety covers over all unused outlets.

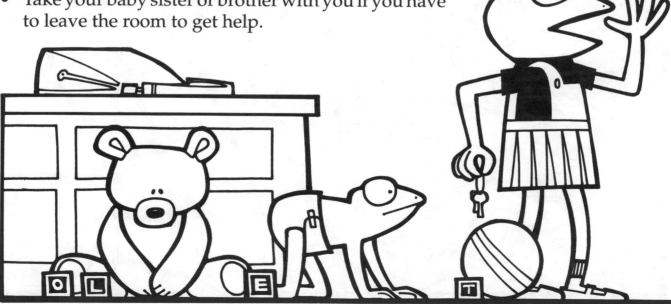

Phone Calls

The telephone rings while your mom
is taking a shower. You answer,
and a person whose voice
you don't recognize asks
if your mother is home.

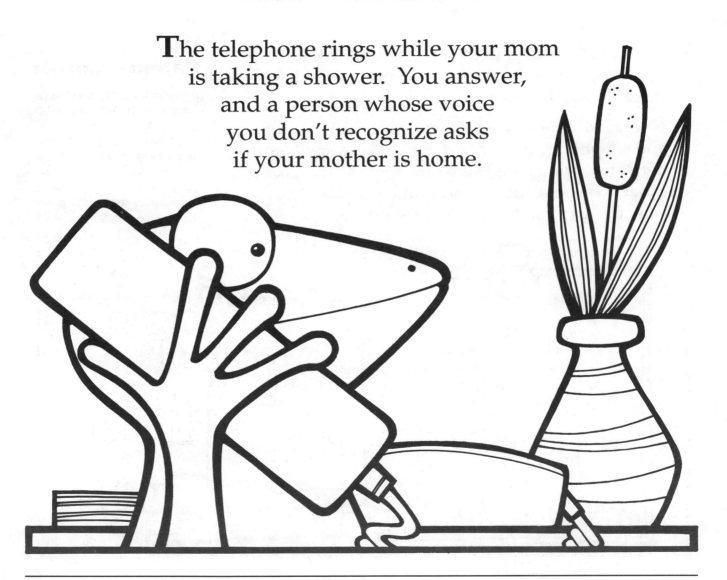

Phone Calls

- Tell the caller that your mom or dad can't come to the phone right now. Ask the person to call back later. Offer to take a message.

- If you take a message, write down the caller's name and telephone number. Ask the caller to spell his or her name if you aren't sure how to write it. Ask the caller to repeat the phone number if you missed something or can't remember the number.

Parents' Corner

Keep a pad of paper and a pencil near the phone so people can take messages.

Show your children where the message pad is and how to use it. Sometimes it helps to pretend you are a caller so your children can practice taking messages.

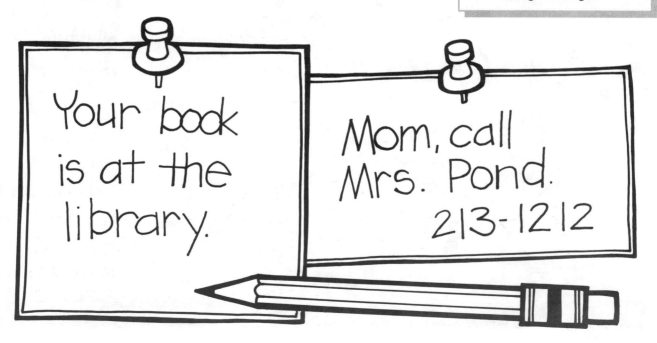

Pills Left on the Counter

One night, when you go to brush your teeth before bed, you find a bottle of pills your grandmother has left on the bathroom counter.

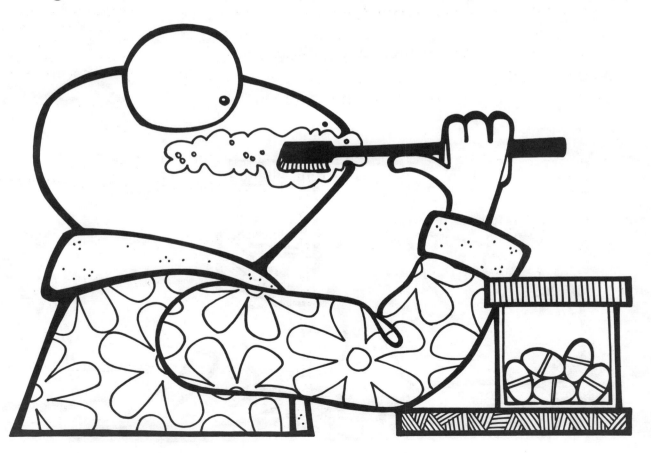

Pills Left on the Counter

- Don't open the bottle of pills.

- Give the bottle to your mom or dad right away.

- Never take medicine that has been prescribed for someone else.

- Never take any kind of medicine without an adult's supervision.

Blackout

You have a baby-sitter for the evening while your parents are out. You and the baby-sitter are reading a story. You're at the best part when the lights suddenly go out. The house is completely dark.

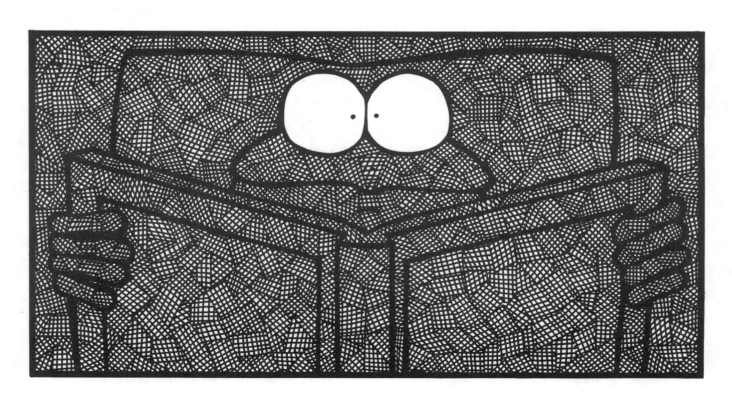

Blackout

- There is no need to get upset. Blackouts are fairly common, especially in and around cities and towns.

- Look out a front window. If every other house or building on your street is dark, the problem is probably a power failure or blackout.

- Wait a few minutes. In most cases, the power comes back on quickly.

- If the power doesn't come back on in a few minutes, tell your baby-sitter where to find a flashlight. Use the flashlight until the lights come back on.

- Don't light candles or matches. Don't use the stairs in the dark.

- If the power stays off for a long time, have your baby-sitter turn on a battery-powered radio and tune in a local station. If the power failure is big enough, you may hear about it on the radio.

Parents' Corner

Keep flashlights handy in several places in your home. Tell your children where the flashlights are kept and demonstrate how to use them. Make sure you have a supply of fresh batteries.

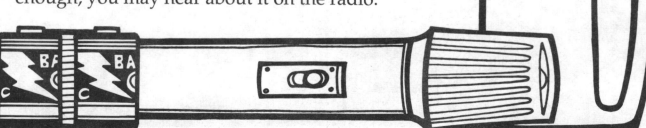

Tub of Water

Your older sister just washed the dog and took him
inside to finish drying him. She left the washtub
in the backyard, and the tub is half full of water.
Your two-year-old brother runs outside to play,
heads straight for the washtub, and bends over
the tub to look inside. Everyone else is in
the house, and your sister doesn't
come when you call her.

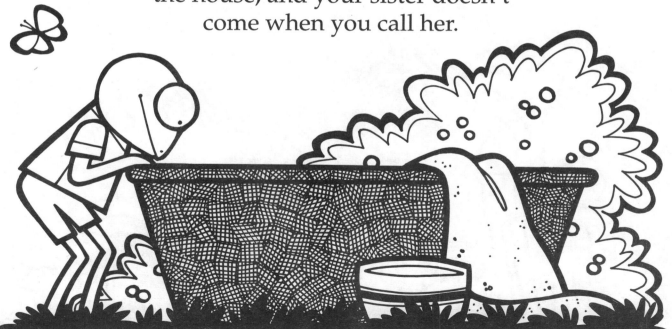

Tub of Water

- Young children can drown in just a few inches of water. They can fall head first into a large bucket or tub and not be able to get out.

- Call for help, or take your brother with you to find your mom or dad. Tell your mom or dad about the tub.

- Make sure the water is poured out or moved to a safe place so no one can fall into it.

Parents' Corner

Always close toilet lids when the toilets aren't being used. This will make it impossible for small children or pets to crawl in and drown.

Check for things with water in them, like diaper pails or laundry tubs. Make sure these containers are out of reach or have tight-fitting lids.

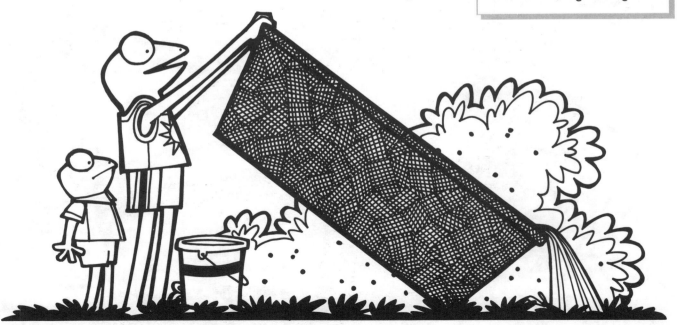

Broken Glass

You are alone in the kitchen after school.
Your mom is upstairs. You want some milk
and decide to get a glass yourself. When you reach
for the glass, you accidentally knock it over.
It shatters all over the kitchen floor.

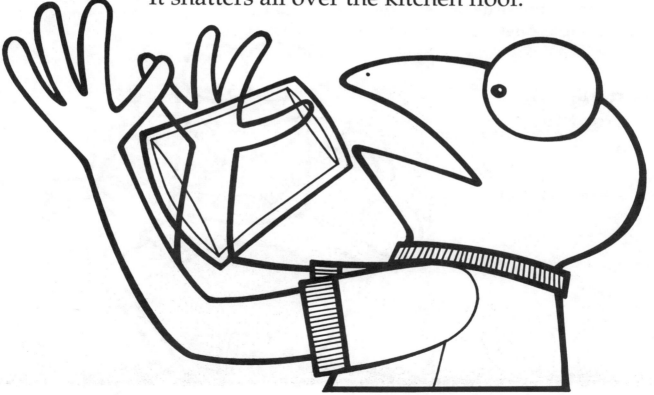

Broken Glass

- Don't touch the broken glass with your hands. You might cut yourself.

- If you're wearing shoes, step carefully around the broken glass. Tell your mom so she can sweep up the glass so that no one gets cut.

- If you're not wearing shoes, don't move. Call your mom and ask her for help.

Parents' Corner

Instead of using a paper towel to pick up small slivers of glass, try using a slice of bread.

Safety Tip for Kids

Use plastic glasses and plates for your after-school snacks. Keep your plastic dishes in a special place that is easy for you to reach.

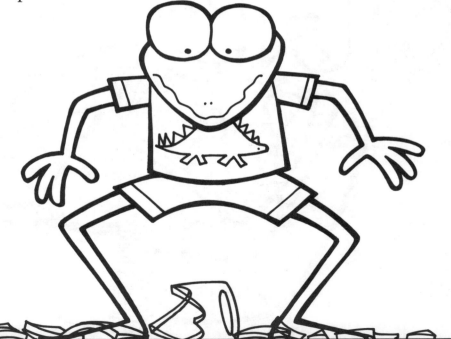

Hot Grill

Your family is having a barbecue in your backyard.
The coals are hot and ready. Your dad goes inside
the house to get the food for the grill. While he
is inside, your cousin begins chasing your dog
around the hot grill.

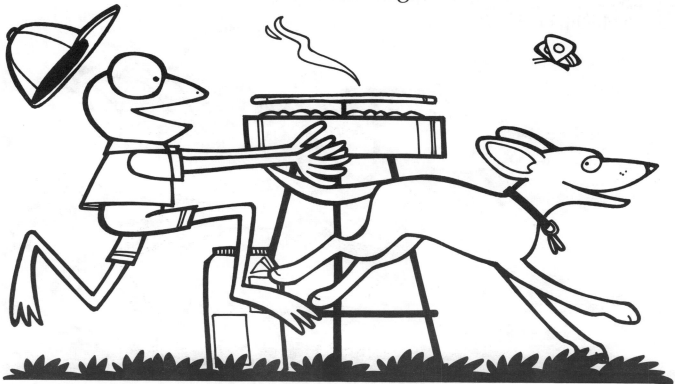

Hot Grill

- It is not safe for anyone to run around a hot grill. People can get burned if they accidentally run into the grill or knock it over.

- Tell an adult so they can supervise your cousin around the hot grill.

- If your dog is excited and running around the grill, tie him up or put him inside the house.

Parents' Corner

Establish a safety zone around the grill. Tell kids to stay at least three feet away. Keep all flammable liquids, such as lighter fluid, away from children.

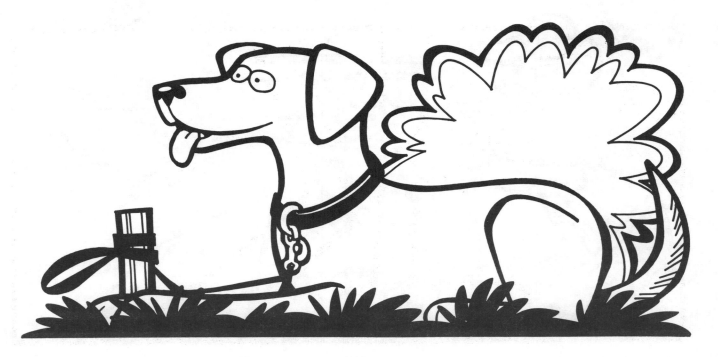

Soap in the Bathtub

You've just finished your bath. Your mom
tells you to get out of the bathtub
and dry yourself. Then the doorbell rings.
She leaves the bathroom to answer the door.
As you stand up, you notice the bar
of soap is sitting on the bottom of the tub.

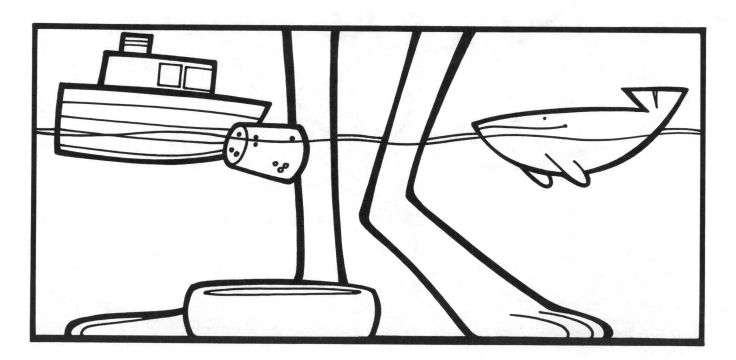

Soap in the Bathtub

- Pick up the soap and put it in the soap holder or soap tray.

- If you leave it there and step on it getting out of the bathtub, you could slip and hurt yourself.

Parents' Corner

Never leave a young child unattended in the bathtub, even for a minute.

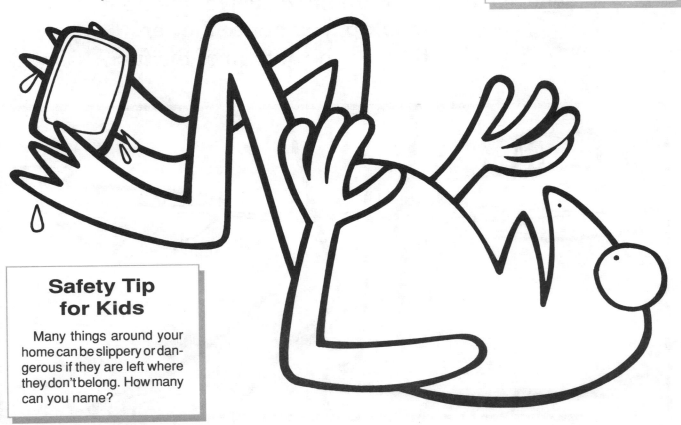

Safety Tip for Kids

Many things around your home can be slippery or dangerous if they are left where they don't belong. How many can you name?

Poisonous Plants

Your dad is cooking dinner and you
are playing with your younger sister to keep
her out of the way. She says, "I'm hungry."
Then she grabs the leaf of a potted plant
and starts to put it in her mouth.

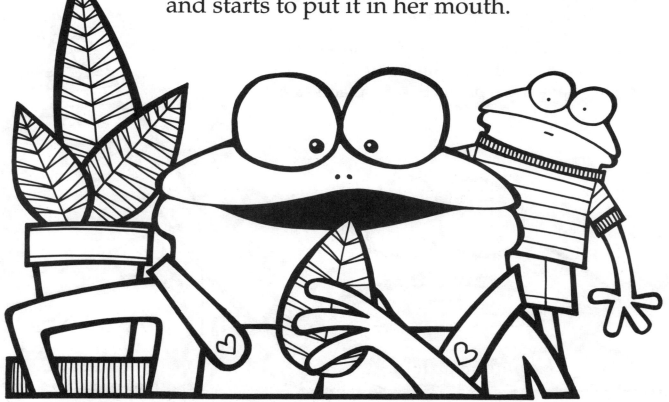

Poisonous Plants

- Take the leaf away from her right away. Many plants are poisonous, and eating them can make people sick.

- Tell your dad what happened.

- You or your dad should move the plant to a place where your sister can't reach it.

- Later, you and your dad can check to see if there are other plants around the house that your sister can reach. Move these plants to safer places, too.

Parents' Corner

See page 183 for a list of common poisonous plants.

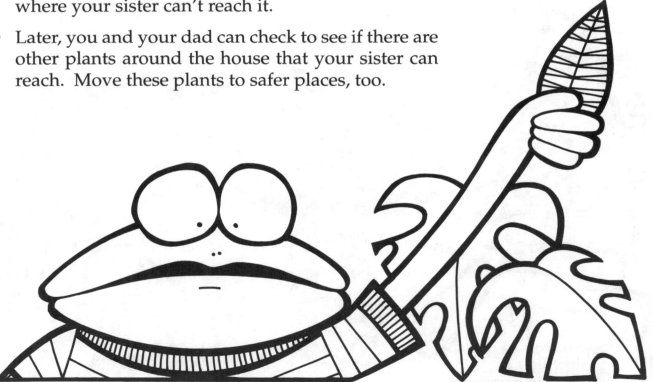

Prowler

It's late at night. A baby-sitter is staying
with you while your mom and dad are out
for the evening. You are in bed, and you think
you hear someone outside your bedroom window.

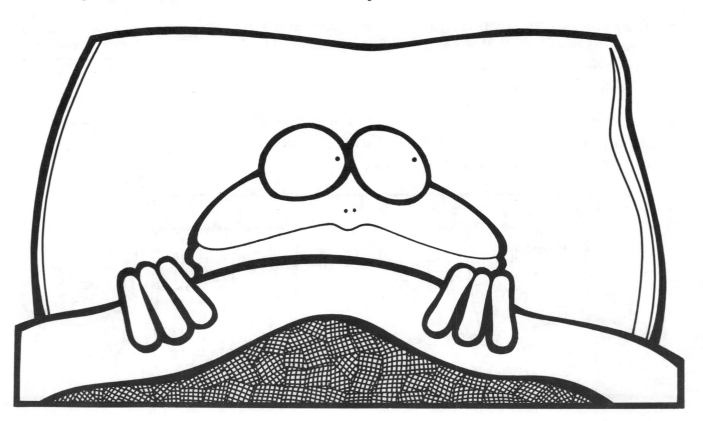

Prowler

- Sometimes the noises you hear outside are made by a dog or the wind rather than by a prowler.

- If you think that there is a prowler outside, tell the baby-sitter right away. The baby-sitter should dial 911.

- Your baby-sitter should check all the doors and windows to make sure they are securely locked. He or she should check those on the ground floor first and pull down or close all blinds, curtains, and drapes.

- Don't go outside or open the door. The baby-sitter should turn on all the outside lights that can be switched on from inside the house.

Parents' Corner

Special motion-detecting security lights are available at most hardware stores. These lights will help you differentiate between the wind and the movement of a body in the yard. Consider installing them outside your home for added safety.

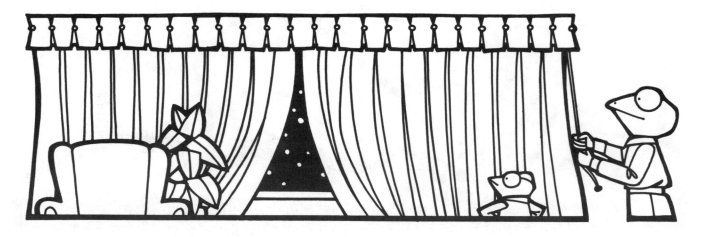

Electrical Fire

Your dad is toasting bread for breakfast.
He runs outside to get the morning newspaper.
While you are eating your breakfast,
a shower of blue sparks and thick smoke
shoots out of the electrical outlet in the wall.

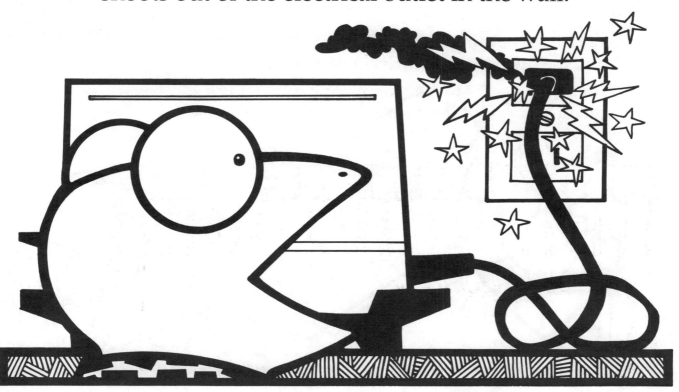

Electrical Fire

- Never throw water on an electrical fire.

- Get out of the kitchen and close the door behind you. Call for your dad.

- If the fire is small and hasn't spread, your dad may be able to put it out with a fire extinguisher.

- If the fire can't be controlled, your dad will dial 911.

- Never enter a burning building. Stay outside and wait for the fire fighters to arrive.

Parents' Corner

Let your children know which appliances they are allowed to use without supervision.

Keep a fire extinguisher in the garage. Be sure that you know how to use it correctly.

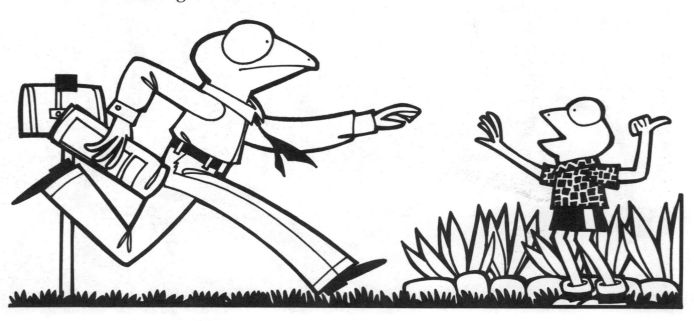

House Fire

During the night, you wake up coughing.
Your eyes burn. You smell smoke.
You call out, but no one answers.
Everyone but you is still asleep.

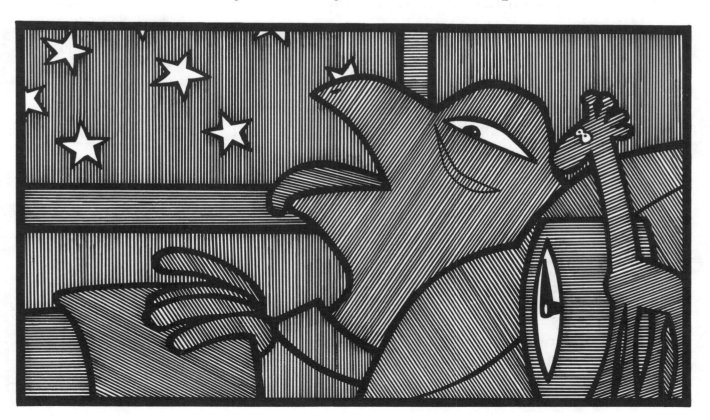

House Fire

- Shout loudly to wake up others.

- If your bedroom door is open and you feel heat or see flames, close the door.

- If your bedroom door is closed, feel the door (not the handle) with your hand. If it is hot, don't open it.

- If your door doesn't feel hot and you don't see flames, leave quickly. Crawl on the floor if there is smoke.

- If you have to wait in your room, shove pillows, sheets, blankets, or clothes in the crack at the bottom of the door to keep smoke out.

- If there is a lot of smoke, tie a scarf or t-shirt over your nose and mouth.

- Don't hide under a bed. Stay by the window so fire fighters can find you quickly.

- If it gets hard to breathe, lie down on the floor. The smoke is usually not as thick there.

- Once you are safely outside, go to your family's meeting spot. After everyone is out safely, send someone to a neighbor's house to call 911.

Parents' Corner

Plan two fire escape routes from each room in your house. Pick a meeting place outside your home where your family can meet after evacuating.

Have fire drills so your children can practice what to do in an emergency.

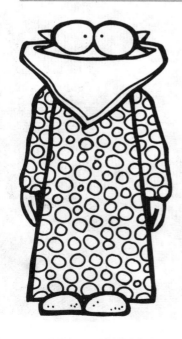

Obscene Phone Call

Just as you are about to go to bed,
the telephone rings. You answer it.
The caller talks about body parts
and uses dirty words.

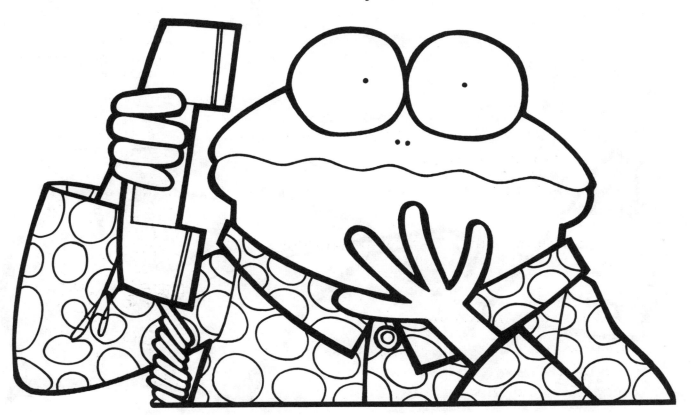

Obscene Phone Call

- Hang up right away. Don't talk to the caller.

- Don't tell the caller who you are, where you live, or what your phone number is.

- Tell your mom or dad about the call as soon as you hang up.

Parents' Corner

If this happens more than once, report the obscene phone calls to the police or the sheriff's department.

Keep a whistle by the phone. Blowing the whistle loudly into the phone can help to discourage the caller from phoning again.

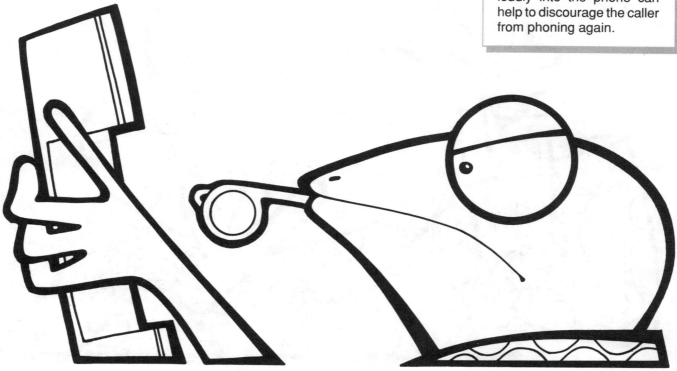

Earthquake

You are setting up a toy dinosaur park in your family room. Suddenly, your dinosaurs fall over and everything starts to shake. You realize that it is an earthquake.

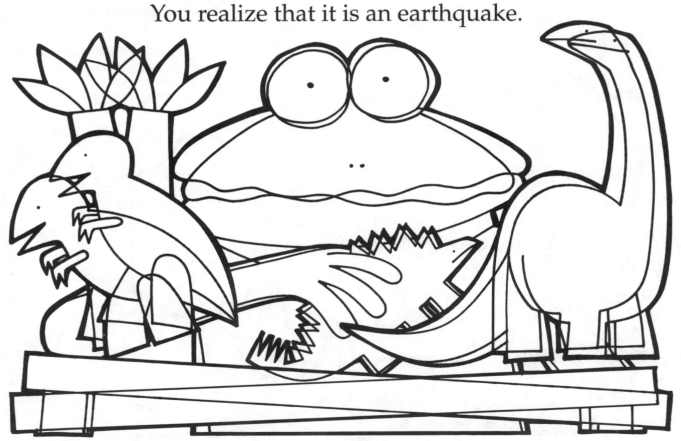

Earthquake

- To avoid being hit by breaking glass and falling objects, stay away from windows and shelves.

- Get under a sturdy desk or table. Hold on to the legs.

- Before you walk around after an earthquake, be sure you have shoes on to protect your feet from broken glass.

- Your parents will check for gas leaks and damage to your home.

- Be aware that earthquakes are frequently followed by smaller earthquakes called "aftershocks."

- After an earthquake or an aftershock, don't open closet or cabinet doors by yourself. Your mom or dad should open them carefully. Things might fall out.

Parents' Corner

See page 188 for a list of equipment and supplies to keep on hand for an earthquake or other emergency.

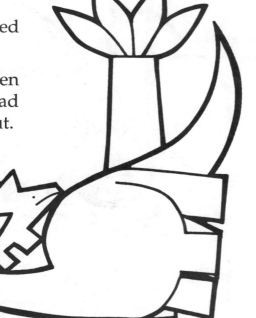

Hurricane

You and your family have been warned
that a hurricane is going to hit
your community within a few hours.

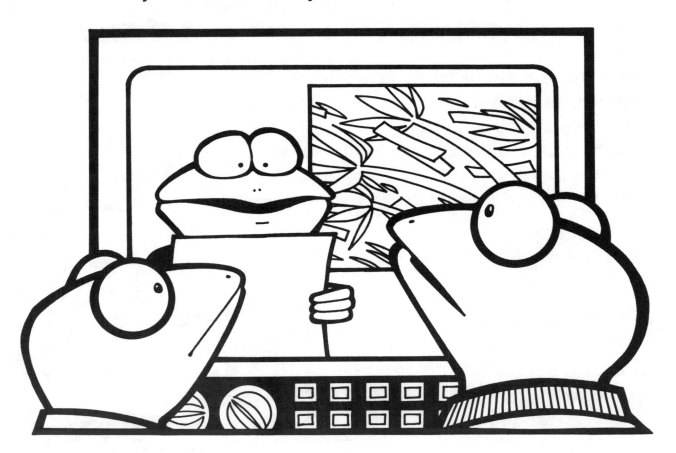

Hurricane

- Help your mom and dad get first aid and emergency supplies together. Fill containers, even bathtubs, with fresh water. Have flashlights, batteries, and a battery-powered radio handy in case the power goes out.

- In a hurricane, the wind and rain stop momentarily, when the "eye," or center, of the storm passes over. Stay inside and away from windows until the entire storm has passed.

- Listen to the radio with your family for weather updates. Don't go outside until the U.S. Weather Bureau reports that the storm is over.

Parents' Corner

Before the hurricane hits your area, close and latch any shutters. Nail sheets of plywood over exposed windows. Check to make sure you have plenty of food and water on hand.

Safety Tips for Kids

When you go outside after the storm, watch for damaged trees that might fall.

Stay away from fallen or low-hanging electrical wires.

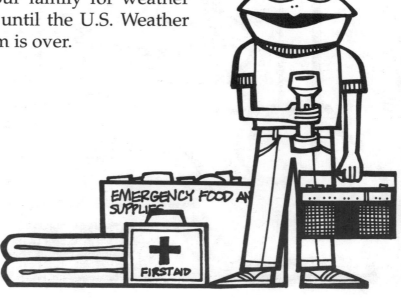

EMERGENCY FOOD AND SUPPLIES

FIRST AID

At School and on the Way

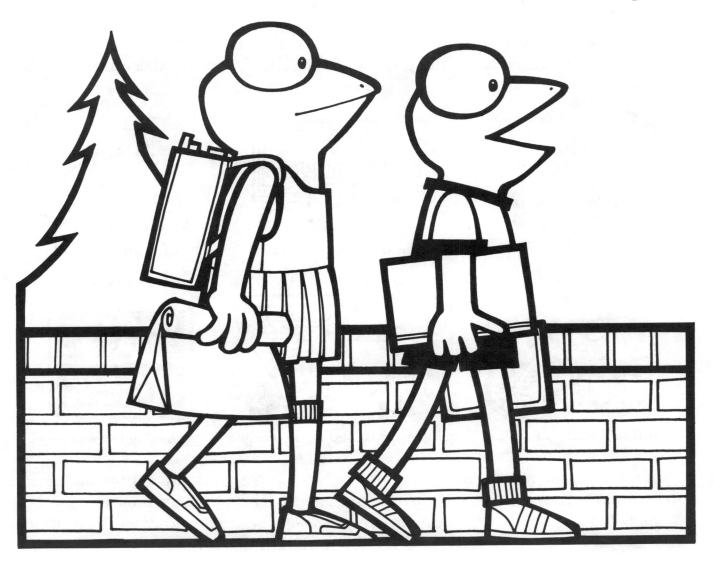

At School and on the Way

In this section, you will find descriptions of situations your child might encounter either at school or while traveling to and from school. Among these situations are

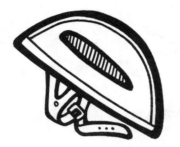

losing a bike helmet

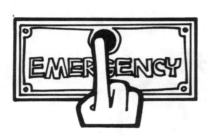

being stuck in an elevator

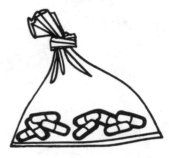

finding a bag of pills

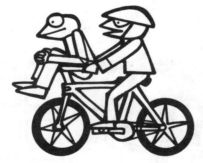

riding double on a bike

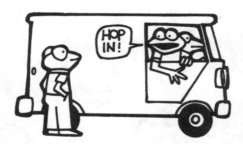

being approached by a stranger

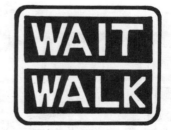

crossing the street

First, read the situation to your child. Next, have your child think about and describe what he or she would do in this situation. Then, turn the page and read the steps listed there to your child. Finally, talk over the steps and discuss additional things you'd want your child to do in this situation.

Parking Lot Problem

Every day, your mom drives you to school
and drops you off in front. Today, as she drives away,
a gust of wind blows your homework out of your hand
and into the school parking lot.

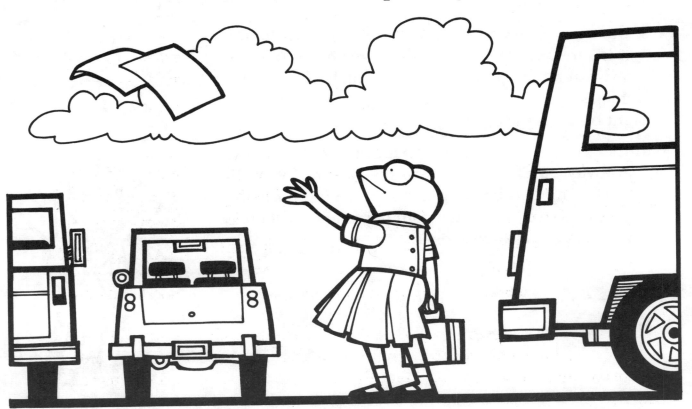

Parking Lot Problem

- Don't run into the parking lot to get your homework. A vehicle might be coming, and you could get hit.

- Look around the parking area for a teacher or another adult. Ask this person to get your paper for you.

- If there's no one you can ask for help, if your homework is in easy reach, and if there are no cars passing nearby, get your paper yourself. Watch carefully for vehicles backing up. Get your homework and get right back on the curb.

- If the wind has blown your paper more than a few feet away, don't chase it across the parking lot. With cars passing and backing up, the parking lot is too dangerous to cross. Leave your paper and explain to your teacher what happened.

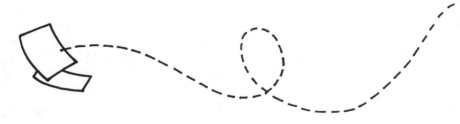
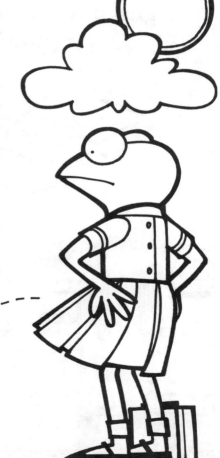

Lost Bike Helmet

The weather is perfect, so you decide
to ride your bike to school. You look
all over the house and garage for
your bike helmet, but you can't find it.

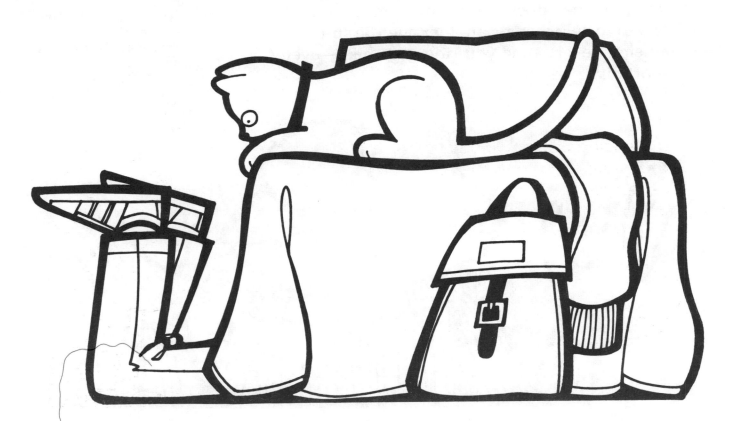

Lost Bike Helmet

- Don't ride your bike **anywhere** without wearing your bike helmet.

- If you cannot find your helmet, walk to school with a group of friends or ask your mom or dad for a ride.

- If your helmet doesn't turn up later, ask your mom or dad to help you get another one. Be sure to wear a helmet every time you ride your bike—even for short distances.

Safety Tips for Kids

For tips on how to find a helmet that is a good fit, see page 193 .

If you are ever in a bike crash, get a new helmet. Your old helmet might have damage you can't see.

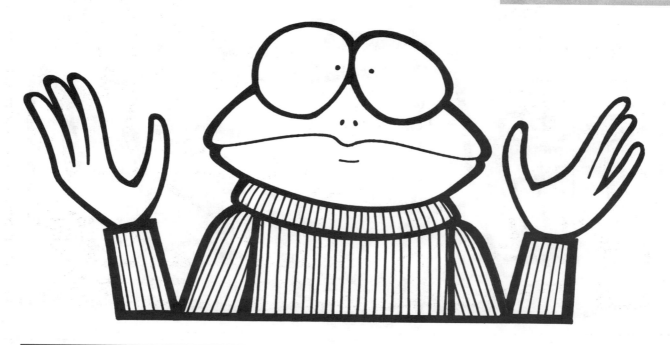

Two on a Bike

You're running to get to school on time.
A friend comes by and offers to give you
a ride on the handlebars of his bike.

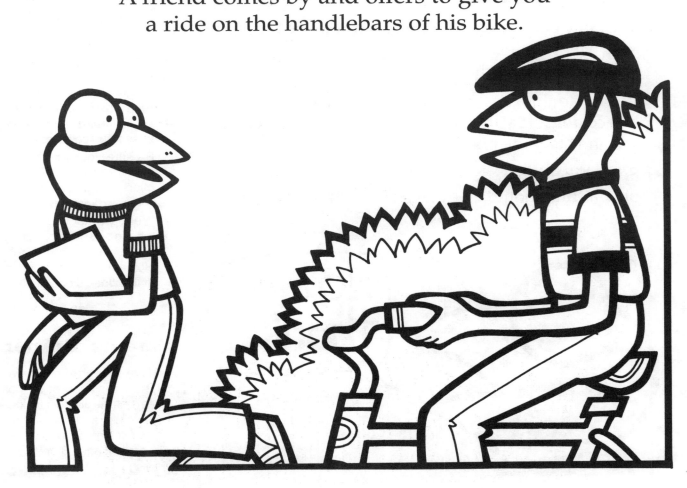

Two on a Bike

- Thank your friend, but don't ride on the handlebars or on the back of anyone's bike.

- Only one person should ride a bike because the only **safe** way to ride a bike is sitting on the bicycle seat, with your feet on the pedals.

- Riding double can throw a bike off balance and cause an accident. It also makes it hard for the "driver" to see and steer the bike.

- Some bikes have special seats for small children, but only adults should ride bikes with small children on board.

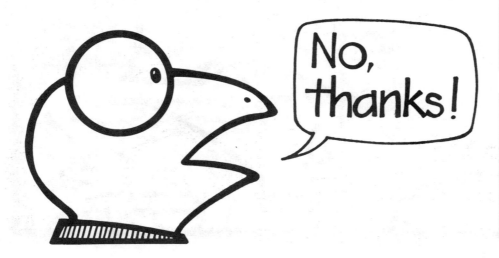

Safety Tips for Kids

If you are old enough to ride in the street, follow these safety tips:

- Ride on the right side of the road, going with the flow of the traffic.
- Stop at all intersections. Walk your bike across busy intersections.
- Be sure your bike is the right size for you. Riding oversized or undersized bikes is dangerous.
- Wear pants with tight legs or use pant clips. Make sure that your clothes can't get caught in the wheels or chain.

Parents' Corner

Have your child ride on a bike path instead of in the street until he or she can ride confidently and follow the basic rules of the road (usually around ages 8 or 9).

Flat Tire

While you are riding to school on your bike,
one of your tires goes flat. Your house is six blocks away,
and you don't want to be late for school.

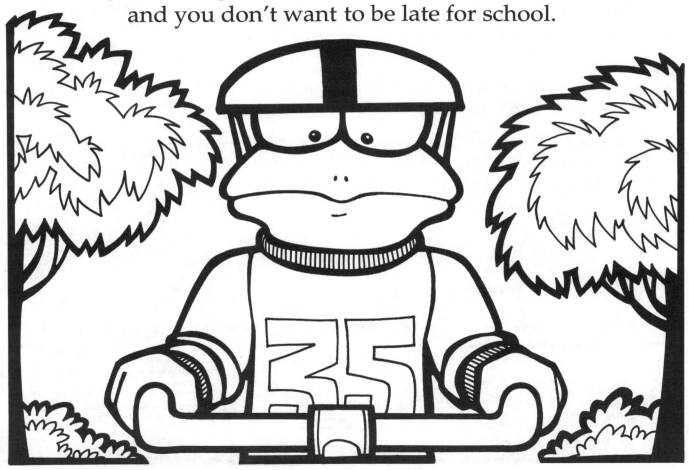

Flat Tire

- If you know people in the neighborhood, ask if you can leave your bike with them for a few hours. Then walk to school.

- If you don't know anyone in the neighborhood, walk your bike to school.

- When you get to school, go to the office and explain why you are late.

- Call your parents and let them know what happened. Tell them where you left your bike. Let them know you will need a ride home after school.

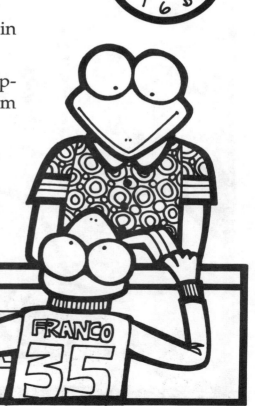

Safety on the Bus

You're riding home on the school bus.
While the bus is moving, you drop your baseball,
and it rolls to the back of the bus. You want
to get out of your seat to get it.

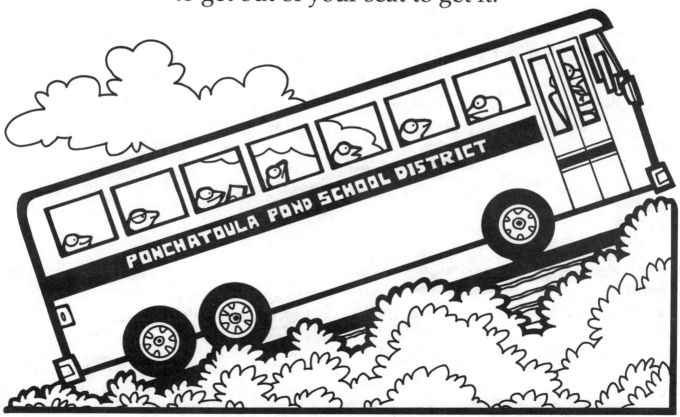

Safety on the Bus

- Stay in your seat. It isn't safe to walk up and down the aisle of the bus while it's moving.

- If the driver makes a sudden stop while you are out of your seat, you could fall and get hurt.

- If the ball stops next to someone on the bus, ask the person to hold it for you until the bus comes to a complete stop and you can get your ball. Be sure to let the driver know what you're doing.

- If the ball rolls to a spot that no one can reach, wait until the bus gets to your stop. Then get your ball.

Safety Tips for Kids

- Get to your bus stop early. Accidents sometimes happen when you are late and run to catch the bus.
- Don't walk behind the bus. Cross the street at least 10 feet in front of the school bus. Sometimes the driver cannot see you if you're closer.

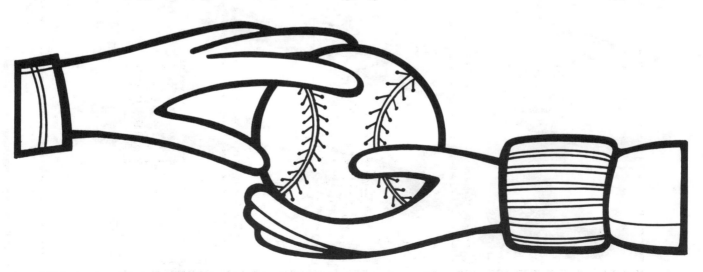

Stuck Elevator

You live on the third floor of an apartment building.
While you are riding the elevator to your apartment
after school, it stops between floors.
No one else is in the elevator.

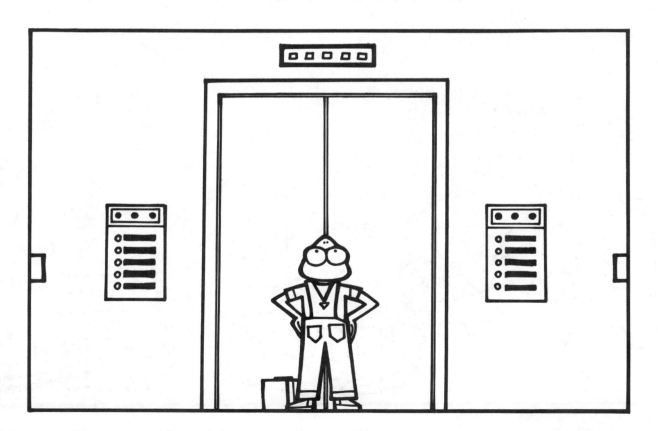

Stuck Elevator

- Wait a minute. The elevator may start up again. If it doesn't, press the "close door" button. Then press the floor button again. (Some buttons need to be pulled out, not pushed in.)

- If the elevator still doesn't move, press the emergency button, which is usually red. An alarm will sound so that other people will know that the elevator is stuck.

- If there is no emergency button or no alarm sounds, stay calm. Attract attention by knocking on the floor, door, or walls. Shout for help. Sooner or later, someone will hear the noise and come to help you.

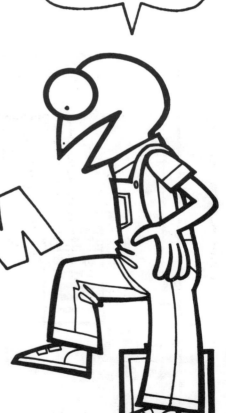

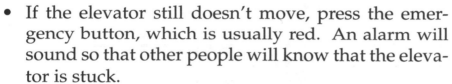

Thrown Objects

When your teacher is out of the room
for a minute, a student starts throwing chalk.
A piece just misses hitting your head.

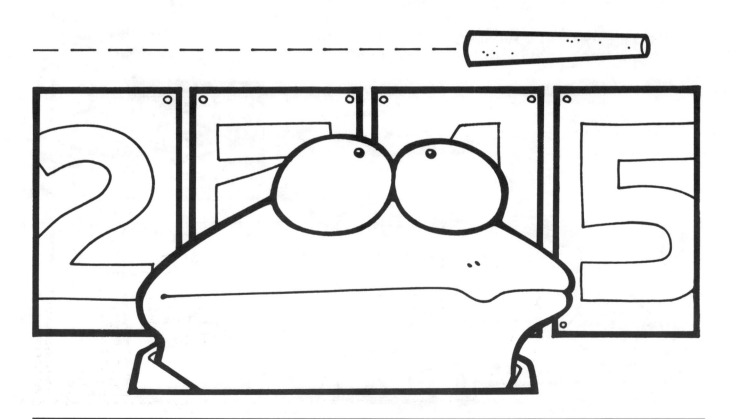

Thrown Objects

- Throwing anything at a person can be dangerous, especially if the object hits someone in the eye.

- Don't throw the chalk or anything else back to the student who threw it . Give it to your teacher or put it back where it belongs after class.

- Tell your teacher what happened so your teacher can explain the dangers of throwing things.

Confused Instructions

While you are in class, you realize that you are confused
about what you are supposed to do after school.
You can't remember if your mom told you to walk home
with your older brother, or wait for her to pick you up.

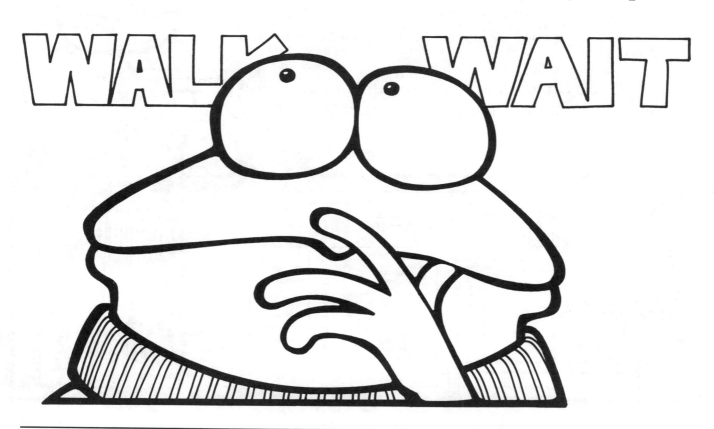

Confused Instructions

- Ask your teacher if you can go to your brother's classroom during lunch or recess to see if he knows what you're supposed to do.

- If your brother is also unclear about your afterschool arrangements, go to the school office and talk to the secretary. Explain that you aren't sure whether you are supposed to walk home after school or wait for a ride.

- Ask if you can use the phone to call your mom and find out what to do when school is out.

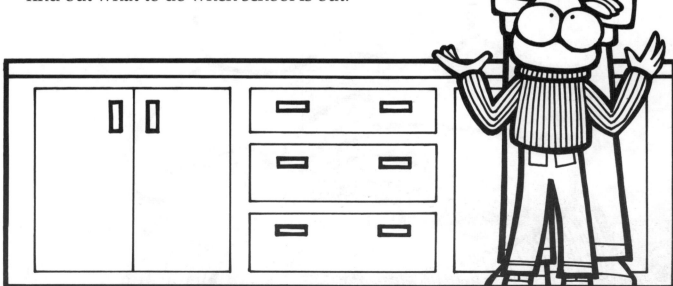

Dangerous Play

On the playground during recess, a friend finds
a large stick and picks it up. She starts
running around, waving the stick.

Dangerous Play

- Tell your friend to stop running with the stick.

- Running with a stick or any sharp object is dangerous. If your friend trips and falls, she could get poked by the stick and seriously hurt. She also might hurt someone else.

- Tell a teacher or playground aide about the situation. The aide will make sure that no one gets hurt with the stick.

Safety Tip for Kids

Besides sticks, what other things can you name that are dangerous to carry when you are running?

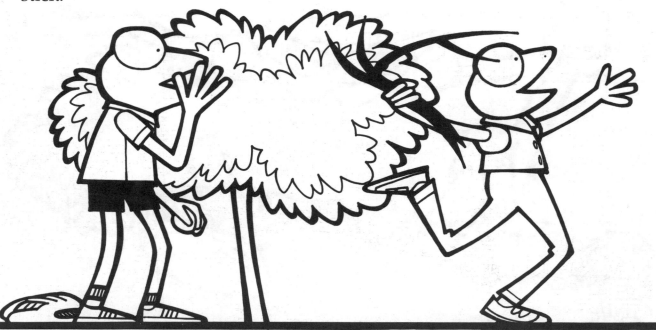

Break-In

One afternoon, your mom meets you at school
and you walk home together. When you get
to your house, the front door is wide open.
No one else is home. Your mom is certain
she locked the door before she left to meet you.

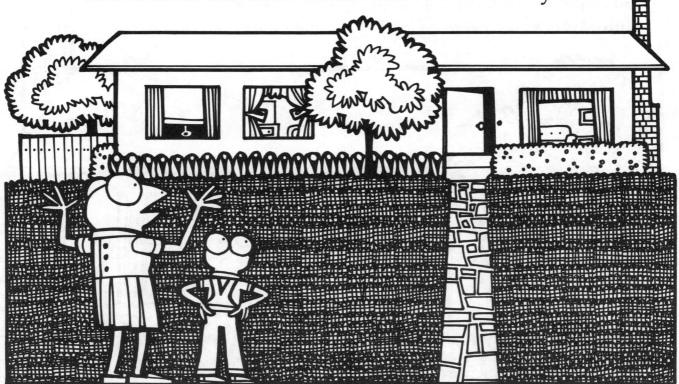

Break-In

- Don't go inside the house.

- Instead, go to a neighbor's or a friend's house with your mom.

- Your mom should dial 911. The operator will send an officer to check inside and outside your house. The police officer or sheriff will make sure it is safe for both of you to go inside.

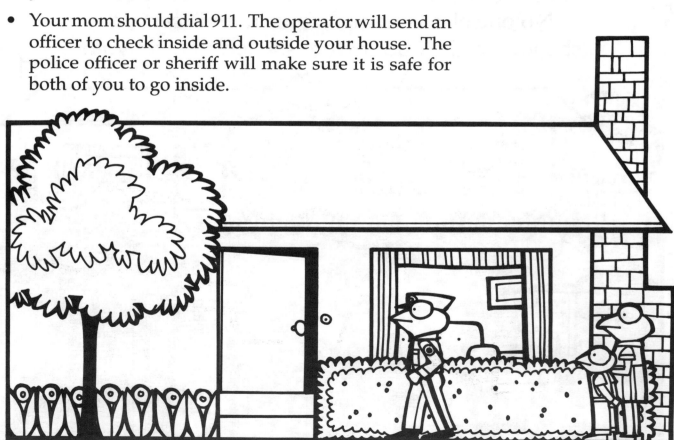

Crosswalk or Jaywalk?

You are walking to school with a friend.
She wants to take a shortcut and cross in the middle
of the block instead of walking to the corner.
She asks you to cross the street with her.

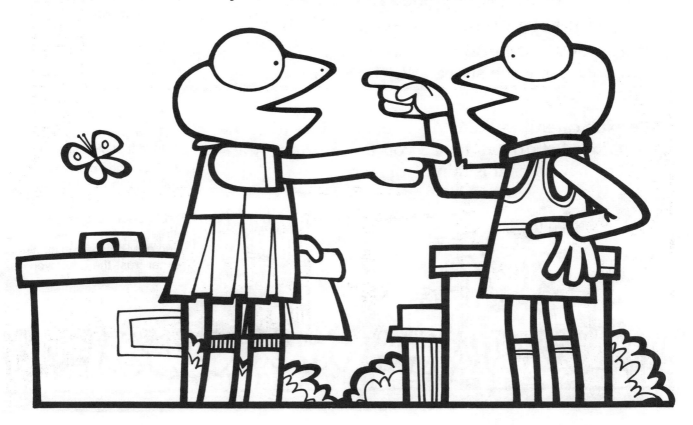

Crosswalk or Jaywalk?

- If you cross in the middle of the block, a driver might not see you or your friend until it is too late to stop.

- Crossing in the middle of the block is called "jay-walking." It's dangerous and often against the law. Tell your friend that you **must** cross at the corner. Ask her to cross with you at the crosswalk.

- When you get to the corner, look both ways for traffic before crossing the street. Watch for cars making turns when you cross.

- Be extra careful walking to school in bad weather. It is harder for drivers to see you and to stop in an emergency when it is raining or stormy.

Parents' Corner

Most kids under age 8 cannot deal safely with traffic for the following reasons:

- They have difficulty discerning which direction sounds are coming from.
- They do not realize that cars can't stop immediately.
- They can't judge how fast traffic is moving.
- Their field of vision is one-third that of adults.
- They often believe that if they can see the driver, the driver sees them.

Practice crossing the street with your child over and over before you let him or her cross the street alone.

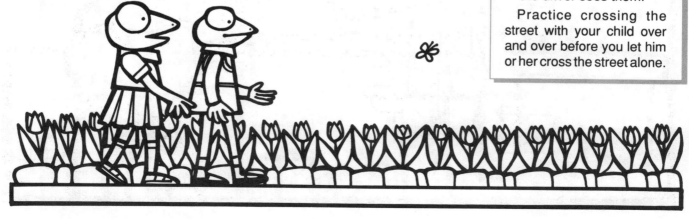

Emergency Pickup

Your friend has a cold, so today you're walking
to school alone. On the way, a stranger comes up to you
and says that your mother has just been hurt
in a car accident. The stranger offers to drive you
to the hospital to see your mother.

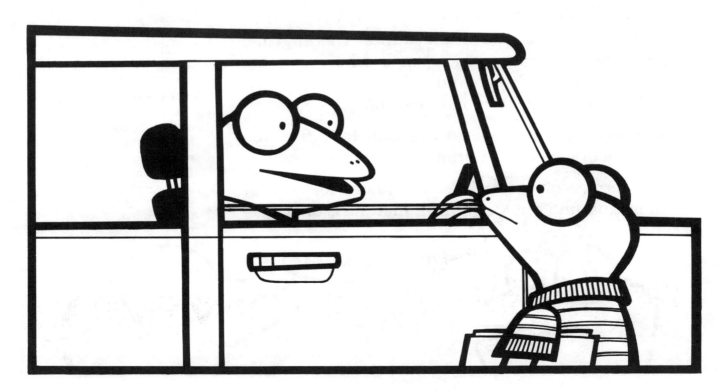

Emergency Pickup

- Don't go! This stranger probably doesn't know anything about your mother and has made up a story to get you into the car.

- Stay out of reach, but try to get a good look at the stranger and the car so you'll be able to tell a police officer what they look like. Try to remember the letters and numbers on the license plate.

- Hurry to the first "safe" adult you see. This might be a neighbor, a police officer, or a school crossing guard. You can also go into a place of business and talk to the person at the cash register.

- When you get to school, go directly to the office. Tell the school secretary or principal what happened.

- Get permission to use the school phone to call your mom and find out for yourself that she is okay.

Parents' Corner

In an emergency, you may need to have your child picked up by someone he or she has not met or may not recognize. To avoid confusion, decide on a secret password with your child. Caution your child to always ask for that password before accepting a ride from a stranger. And remember to tell any authorized emergency driver the secret word!

Don't let your child wear clothes or carry items with his or her name printed large enough for others to read. Children are easily confused when strangers call them by name.

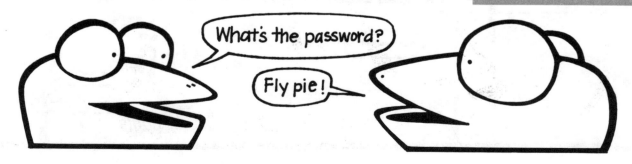

What's the password?

Fly pie!

Bag of Pills

When you go out for recess,
you find a small plastic bag of pills
on the school playground.

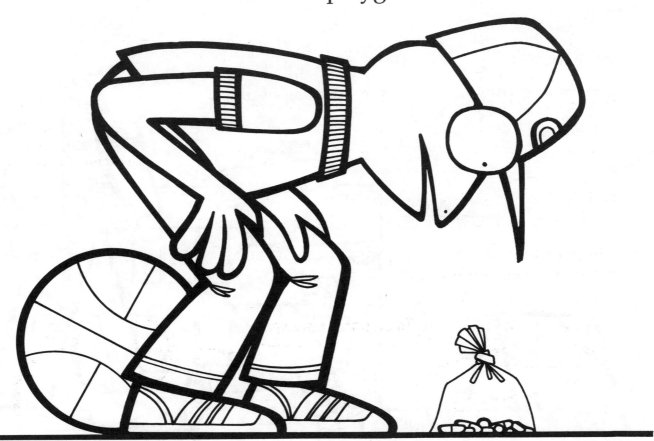

Bag of Pills

- Don't touch the bag.

- Ask two of your friends to watch the bag while you go get an adult. Tell them not to touch the bag or open it.

- Tell the school playground aide, a teacher, a school secretary, or the principal right away.

- Show the adult where you found the bag of pills.

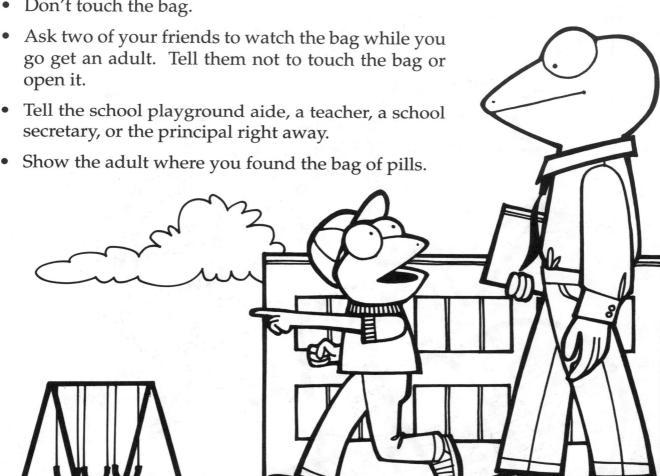

At Play

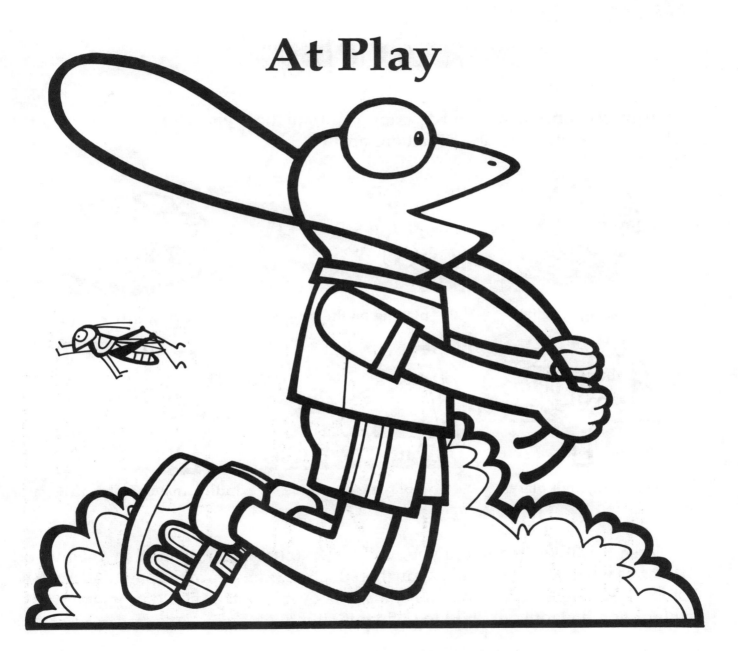

At Play

In this section, you will find descriptions of situations your child might encounter while at play. Among these situations are

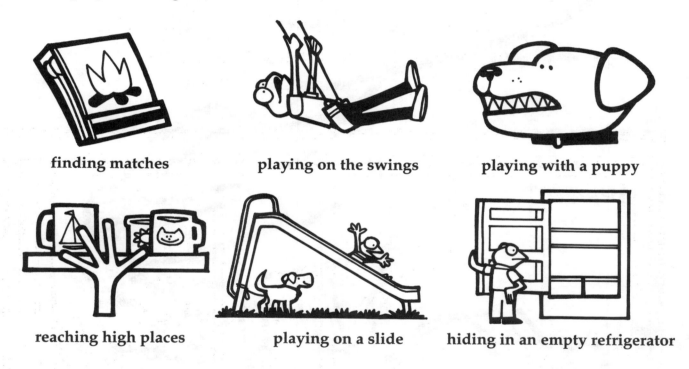

finding matches **playing on the swings** **playing with a puppy**

reaching high places **playing on a slide** **hiding in an empty refrigerator**

First, read the situation to your child. Next, have your child think about and describe what he or she would do in this situation. Then, turn the page and read the steps listed there to your child. Finally, talk over the steps and discuss additional things you'd want your child to do in this situation.

Sliding Glass Doors

Mom and Dad have invited your neighbors over
for a pizza dinner. While the grown-ups
are busy talking in another room, the kids
are running in and out of the house
through a sliding glass door.

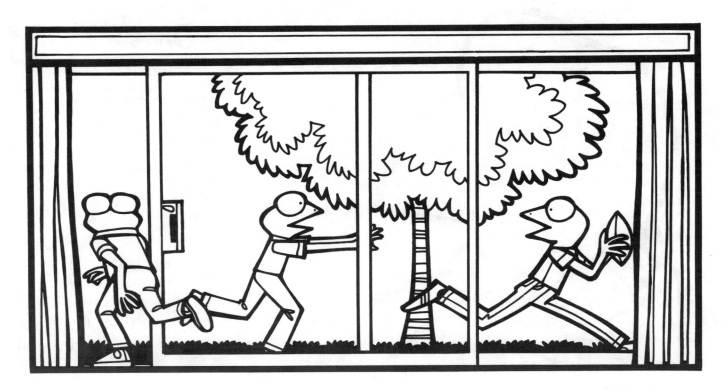

Sliding Glass Doors

- Tell an adult. If the kids run into the glass door while it's closed, they can get a bad bump on the head or cut themselves if the glass breaks.

- Sometimes it's hard to tell if a glass door is open or closed. Always check to be sure a sliding glass door is **open** before going in or out.

Parents' Corner

Try suggesting another activity the kids can all do together that will take them away from the glass door.

Decals for glass doors are available in many hardware stores. These decals serve as good reminders for all family members that a glass door is closed.

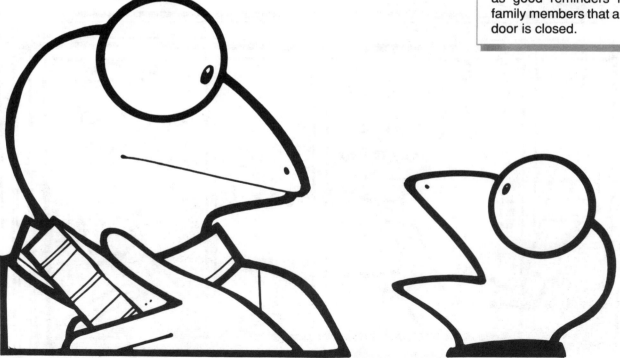

Matches

You are at a friend's house after school.
Your friend finds matches in a kitchen drawer
and asks if you want to play with them.

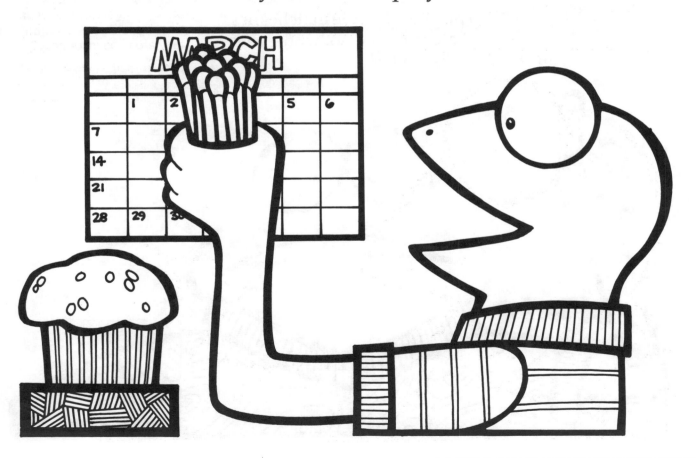

Matches

- Tell your friend you don't play with matches.

- Tell your friend to put the matches back where they were.

- If your friend insists on playing with the matches, let an adult know immediately before someone gets burned or your friend causes a fire.

Safety Tip for Kids

Besides matches, what other things around your house could cause a fire if they are used incorrectly?

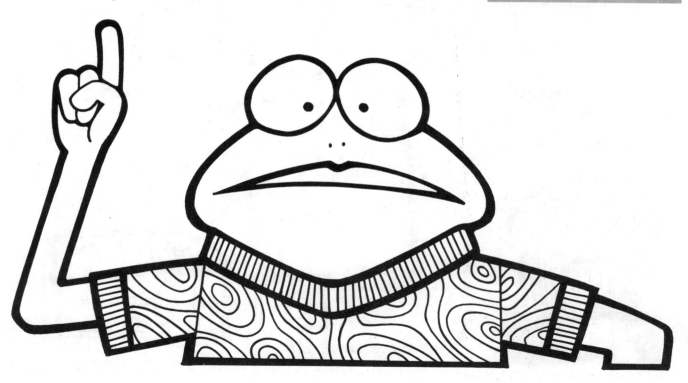

Small Toys and Small Children

Your baby brother is sitting on the floor in your bedroom
watching you play with your toys. All of a sudden,
you see him grab a small piece from your
plastic building set and start to put it in his mouth.

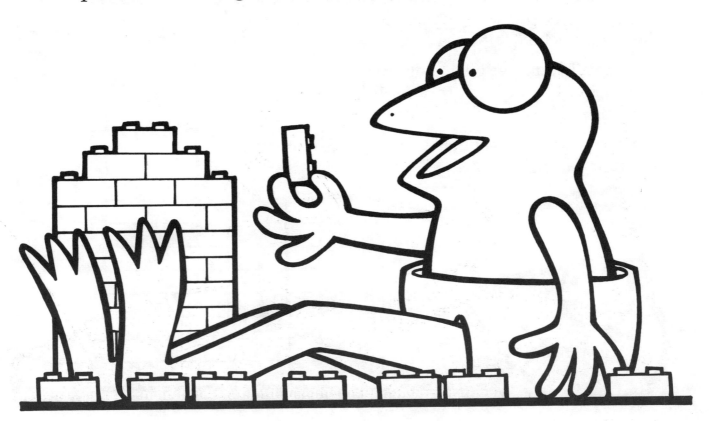

Small Toys and Small Children

- Take the toy away from him at once and put it out of his reach. A young child can easily choke on a small toy.

- If a younger brother or sister is going to be with you when you play with small toys, be sure he or she is in a playpen, or put your toys on a table where they can't be reached.

- Pick up all your toys when you are finished playing. Put them in a safe place, out of the reach of young children.

- If a child actually swallows a toy, get help from your mom or dad right away.

Parents' Corner

See page 191 for instructions on helping a person who is choking.

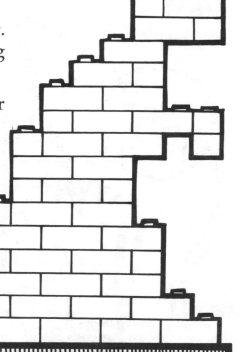

Things in High Places

The board game you want to play
with your friend is on the top shelf of your closet.
Your friend wants you to reach it by standing
on books piled on a chair.

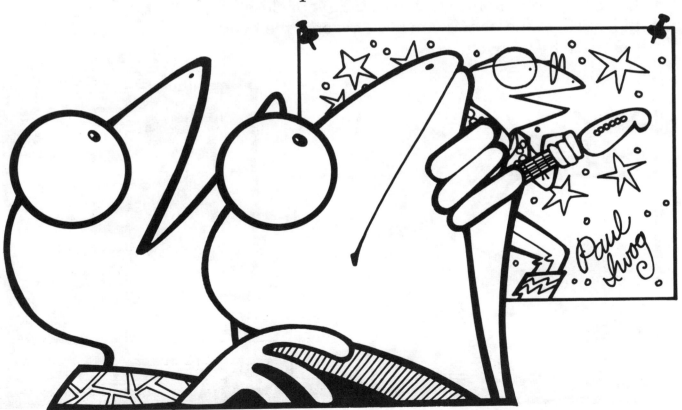

Things in High Places

- Don't pile items on a chair and stand on the pile to reach toys or anything else. You could easily fall and get hurt.

- Ask your mom or dad to get the game for you.

- Later, help your mom or dad rearrange your closet so that the toys and games you need are on a shelf you can reach by yourself.

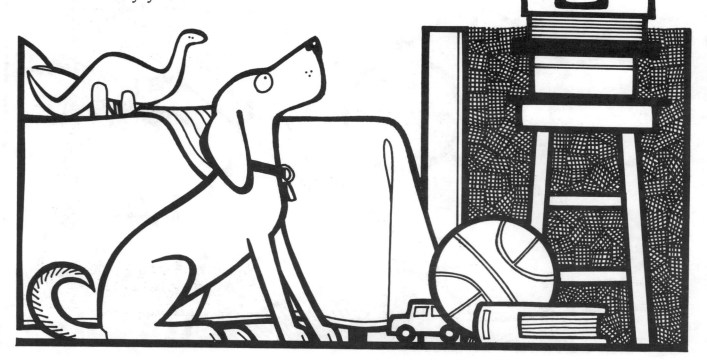

Safety on the Slide

You are playing on a slide in the park.
When you reach the top and are ready to slide down,
you see a young child playing in the sand
at the bottom of the slide.

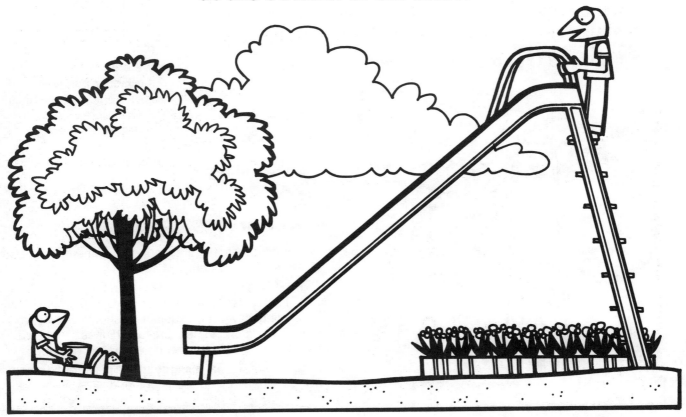

Safety on the Slide

- Don't go down the slide until it is clear below!

- Ask the child to please move out of the way and play in an area away from the slide.

- Tell the child that someone coming down the slide can crash into a kid at the bottom and both kids could get hurt.

- Ask an adult for help if you need it.

Safety Tips for Kids

- Always sit down and face forward when you go down the slide. Never go backwards or stand up while going down the ramp.

- If there's a line, stay on the ladder and wait until the kid ahead of you goes down before you sit down on the slide.

- Don't push or shove other kids in line or on the slide.

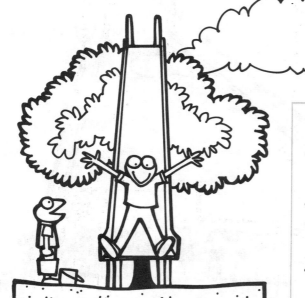

Parents' Corner

- Before your child uses the playground equipment, check to make sure that the equipment is of a size that cannot trap your child's body or head.

- Kids can be injured if they fall off playground equipment. The area surrounding playground equipment should be relatively soft to cushion falls and to help prevent injuries. Avoid playground equipment that is located on asphalt or cement.

- Discourage your child from doing stunts on playground equipment. Don't let them run up slides or stand while swinging.

Discarded Refrigerator

You are playing at a friend's house. You both go
into the garage to get a soccer ball, and you find an
old, empty refrigerator that isn't working.
Your friend suggests that you pretend the refrigerator
is your fort instead of playing ball.

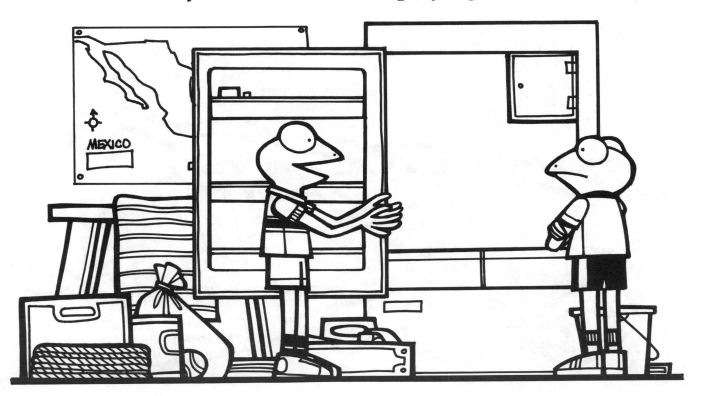

Discarded Refrigerator

- Do **not** hide in a refrigerator or use it in play. Tell your friend not to get in either.

- If you play in a refrigerator and the door closes, you could get locked in. You would quickly run out of air to breathe. You could suffocate.

- When you get home, tell your mom or dad about the refrigerator at your friend's house. Your parents may want to call your friend's parents and suggest that a lock be put on the refrigerator door or that the door be removed so kids can't climb inside and get trapped.

Parents' Corner

Many kids enjoy hiding in small, out-of-the-way places. Explain the dangers, such as suffocation or a cave-in. Check your house, yard, and neighborhood play areas for potentially dangerous spots.

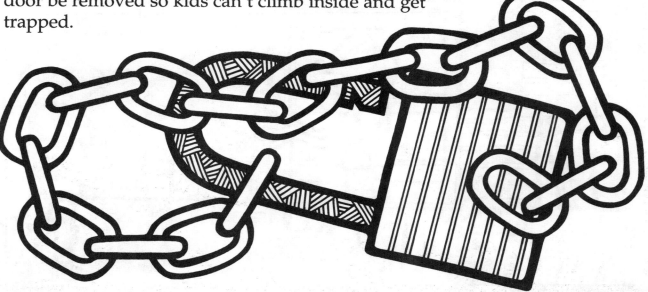

Playing With a Puppy

You want to play with your new puppy,
but she has just started to eat her dinner.
When you reach for her, she growls at you.

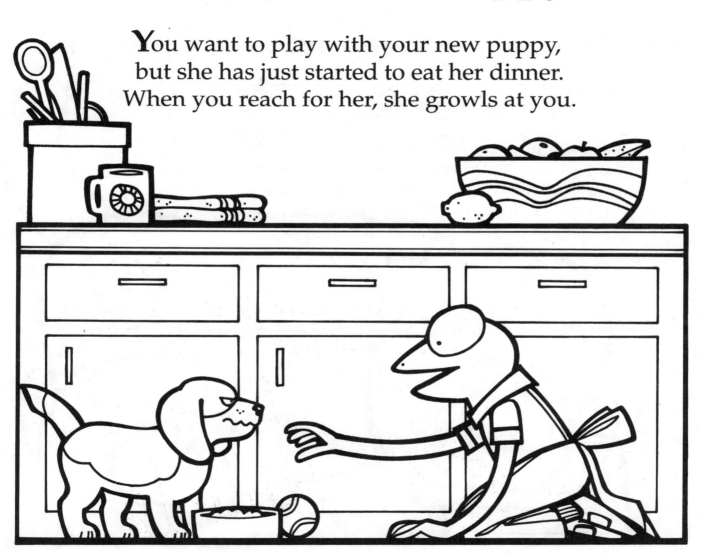

Playing With a Puppy

- Never disturb a pet that is eating or sleeping.

- When your puppy is hungry, she doesn't want to play. She might bite you to get you to leave her alone.

- Wait until your puppy has finished eating. Then have fun playing together.

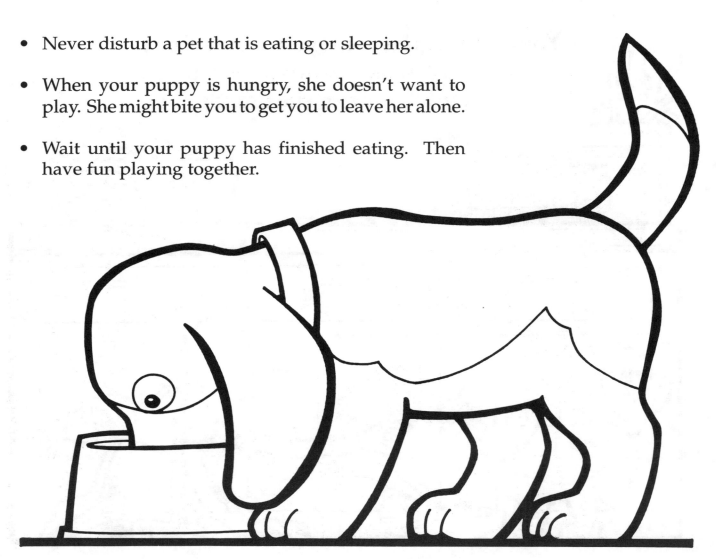

Games on the Stairs

You are visiting your cousin, who lives in a two-story house. She wants to play tag up and down the stairs.

Games on the Stairs

- Stairs are not a safe place to play.

- You can get badly hurt if you trip and fall down the stairs. You can break your arm or leg, or you can hit your head.

- When you walk up or down stairs, hold on to the railing.

Parents' Corner

Install a gate or guard rail across the stairs if you have toddlers.

Safety Tips for Kids

- Always walk up and down the stairs—never run.

- Take one step at a time—not two or three.

- Don't leave toys on the stairs. Someone might trip on them and fall.

- Never push or shove anyone on the stairs.

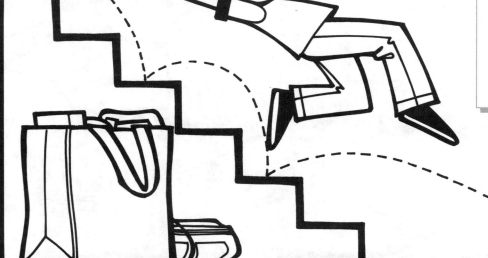

Safety on the Swings

You are playing on the swings at school.
All of a sudden, a classmate comes up behind you
and starts to push you higher and higher. The swing
feels out of control, and you are afraid you're going to fall off.

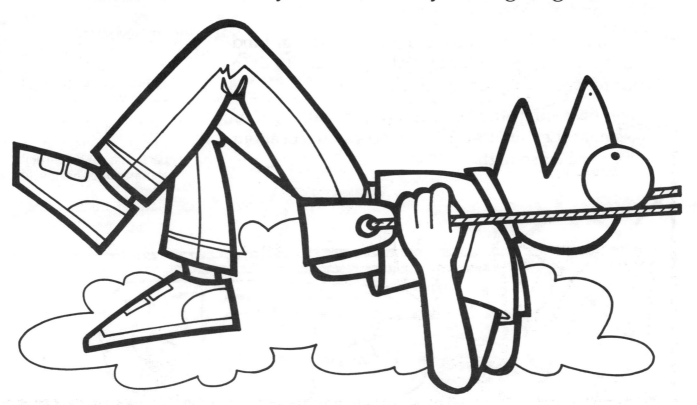

Safety on the Swings

- Tell your classmate to stop pushing right away.

- If you're being pushed too high and your friend won't listen, call an adult for help.

- Stop pumping with your legs so the swing will slow down and you can get it under control.

- You can also drag your feet lightly on the ground each time you swing backward. Don't try to drag your feet when you are going forward.

- When the swing stops and you get off, talk to your classmate. Let him or her know how you feel about being pushed so high.

Safety Tips for Kids

- Always stay seated while swinging. Standing up on a swing is dangerous.

- Swing in a straight line, not crooked or twisted.

- You can get hurt if you're hit or knocked down by someone in a swing. If you're waiting your turn, stand a safe distance back. Wait until the swing stops completely and the person leaves before getting on and beginning your turn.

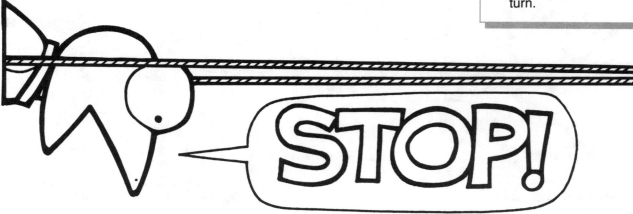

Unsafe Pool Play

Four of your friends have come to your house
to swim in your pool one weekend. Your mom
will be watching you, but first she has to go
in the house to move the phone outside. She tells
everyone to stay out of the pool until she gets back.
While she is inside, one of the kids starts trying
to push the others into the pool.

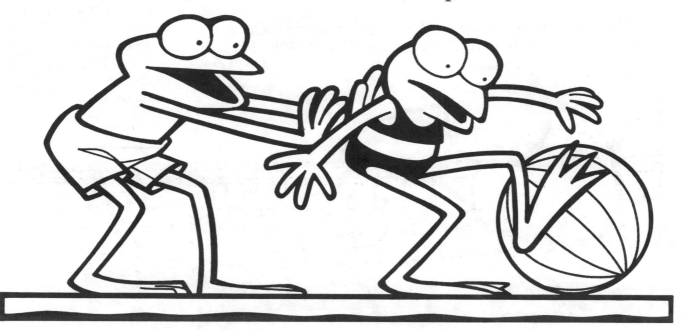

Unsafe Pool Play

- Call your mom right away! If she doesn't hear you, go inside and let her know what is happening before someone gets hurt.

- When you're pushed into a pool, you can bump your head on the side or hurt others if you land on them. Someone might drown.

Safety Tips for Kids

- Never go into the pool alone. Make sure an adult is watching you.

- Always walk around a pool—don't run.

- Don't go into the deep end of the pool unless you have permission from an adult and you know how to swim.

- Don't dive into the shallow end of the pool.

What other swimming pool safety rules do you know?

Parents' Corner

Never leave a child unattended at a swimming pool, even for a moment.

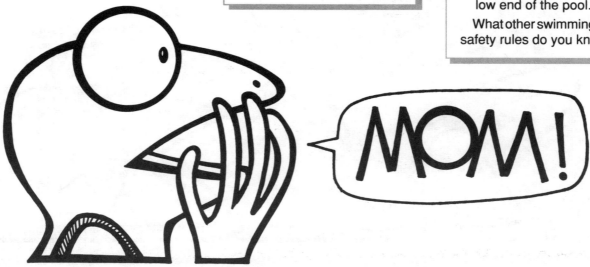

Stray Dog

While you're playing in front of your house
with your friends, a stray dog wanders into the yard.
One of your friends runs over to pet the dog.

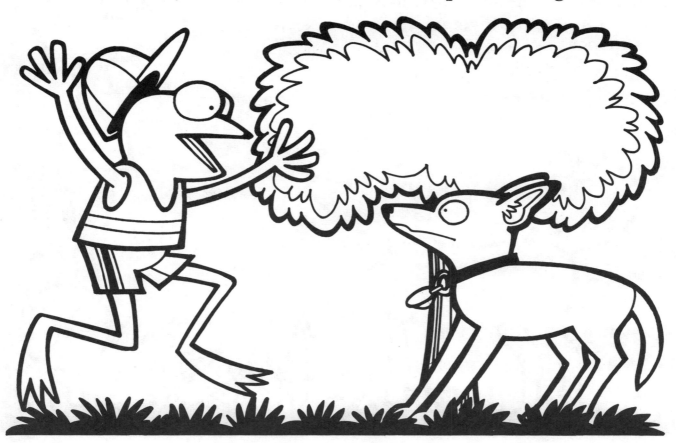

Stray Dog

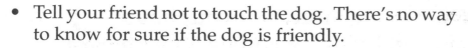

- Tell your friend not to touch the dog. There's no way to know for sure if the dog is friendly.

- Even dogs that are usually friendly may growl or bite if they are tired, hungry, or scared. Leave a dog alone if it growls or tries to get away from you. Never chase a strange dog.

- Tell your dad or mom about the dog. If the dog is wearing a license or I.D. tags, an adult can call the dog's owner or your local animal shelter.

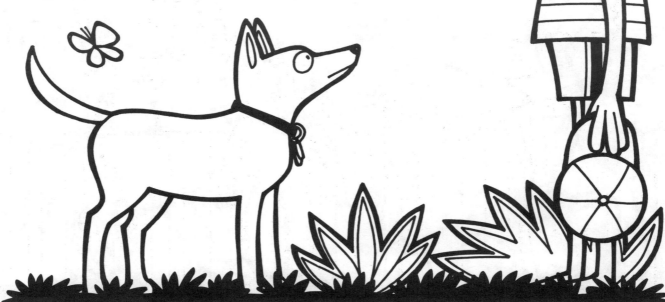

Ball in the Street

You and your friends are playing catch in your front yard.
Someone makes a wild throw, and the ball flies out
an open gate. It bounces and rolls right into
the middle of the street.

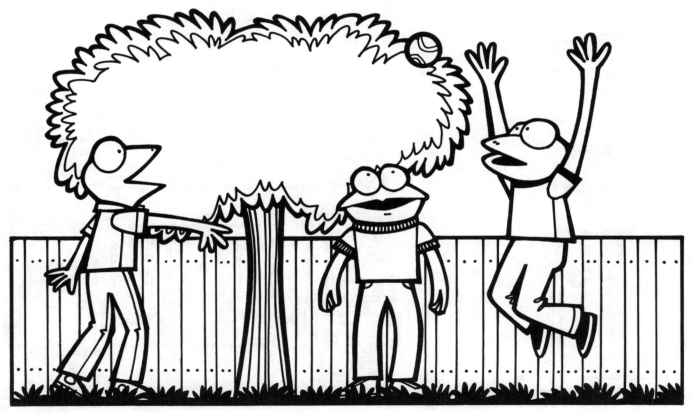

Ball in the Street

- Don't run into the street after the ball. In your excitement to get the ball, you might forget to watch for traffic.

- Ask your mom or dad to get the ball for you.

- Watch how he or she looks both ways for traffic before going into the street for the ball.

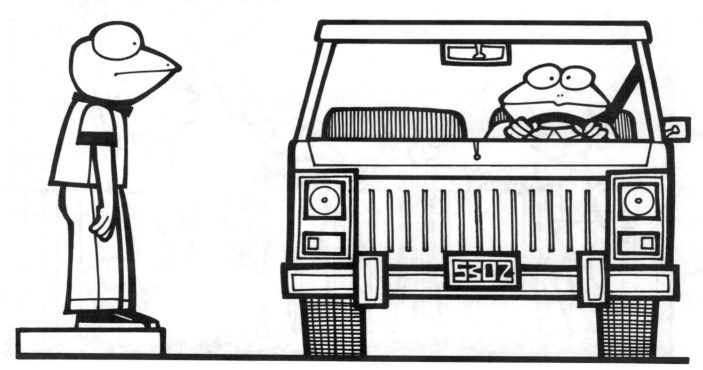

Out and About

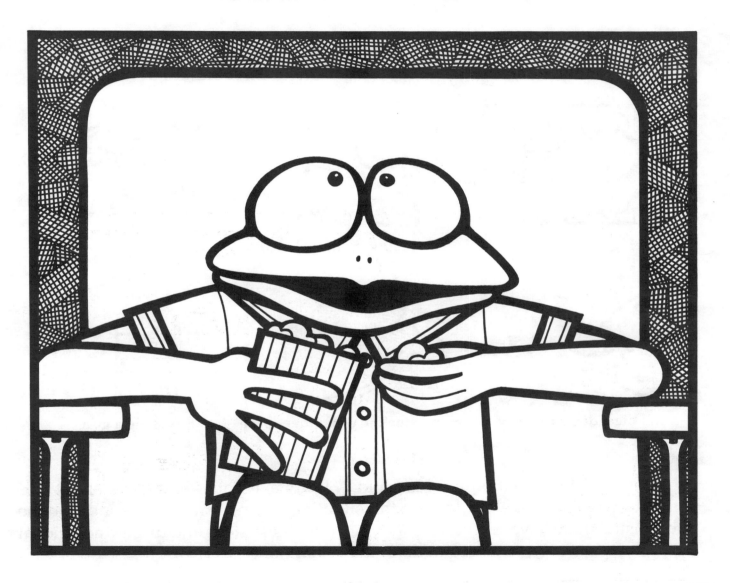

Out and About

In this section, you will find descriptions of situations your child might encounter while out and about in the neighborhood. Among these situations are

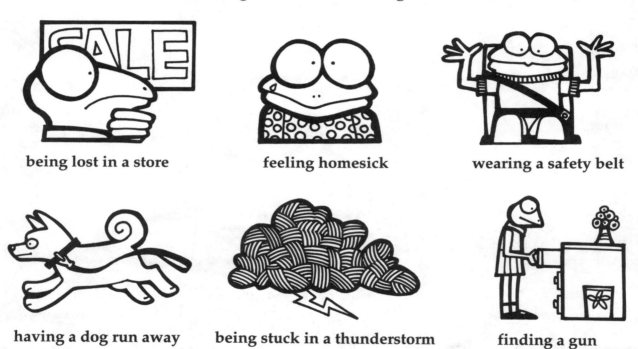

being lost in a store   **feeling homesick**   **wearing a safety belt**

having a dog run away   **being stuck in a thunderstorm**   **finding a gun**

First, read the situation to your child. Next, have your child think about and describe what he or she would do in this situation. Then, turn the page and read the steps listed there to your child. Finally, talk over these steps and discuss additional things you'd want your child to do in this situation.

Plastic Bags

You and your younger sister are with your mom
at the supermarket. Your sister is riding in the seat
of the grocery cart. While your mom is busy
picking out fruit, your sister grabs a plastic bag
and starts to put it over her head.

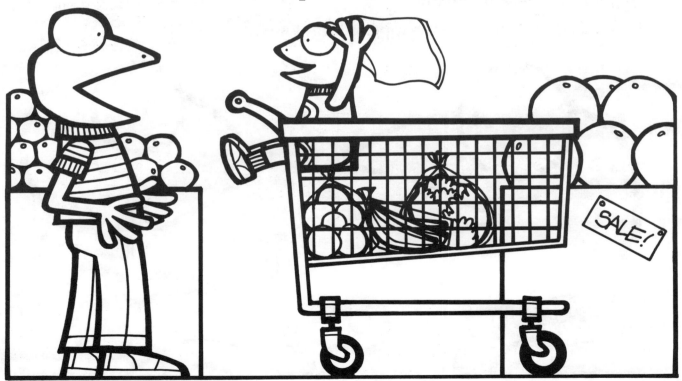

Plastic Bags

- Take the bag away from your sister immediately!

- Move the shopping cart so she can't reach any more bags.

- Tell your sister it's dangerous to put **any** plastic bag over her head. The bag can stick to her face, and she might not be able to breathe.

- Let your mom know what happened right away.

Parents' Corner

Keep the plastic bags that laundry and dry cleaning come in away from your children. These bags should be cut up or tied in knots immediately to avoid an accidental suffocation.

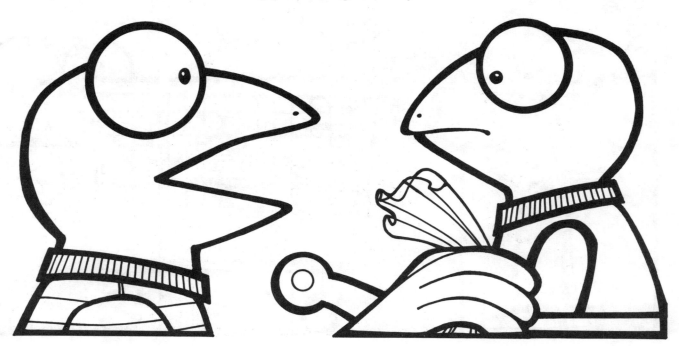

Runaway Pet

When you are walking your dog, he sees a cat across the street. He dashes into the street after the cat, pulling the leash from your hand.

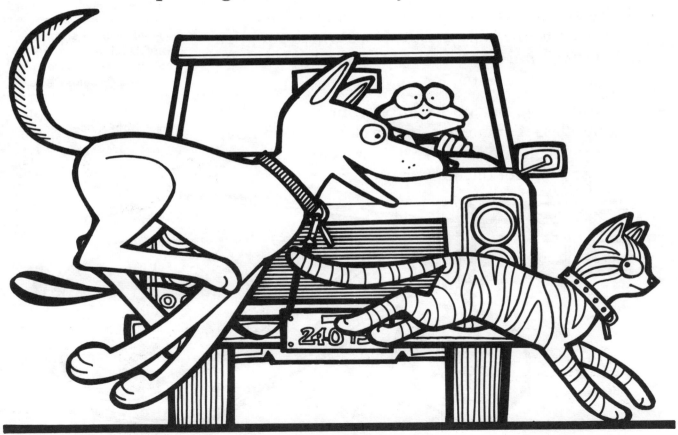

Runaway Pet

- Don't run into the street after your dog.

- Call your dog's name to see if he will come back to you.

- If your dog doesn't come back, go home. Ask one of your parents to take you to the place where your pet ran away. Bring along a treat for your dog, and call his name as you search.

- Ask your mom or dad to enroll your pet in a dog training class. For information on classes, your mom or dad can call your local YMCA, recreation department, or chamber of commerce.

Parents' Corner

Animal control officers are often unable to locate pet owners because the animals aren't wearing adequate identification. For your pet's protection, license the animal and place an identification tag on your pet's collar. Be sure that your dog or cat is wearing the collar and tags every time it goes outside.

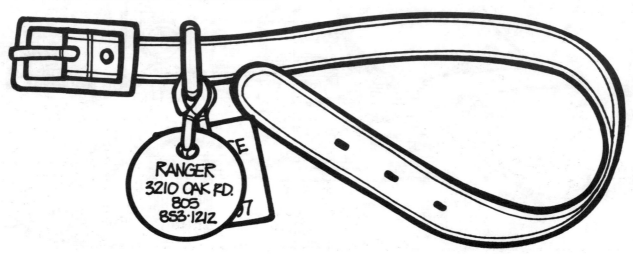

Lost in a Store

One afternoon, your dad takes you
to the sporting goods store. You're busy
checking out the new bikes, until you realize
you can't see your dad anywhere. You look
up and down the aisles, but you can't find him.

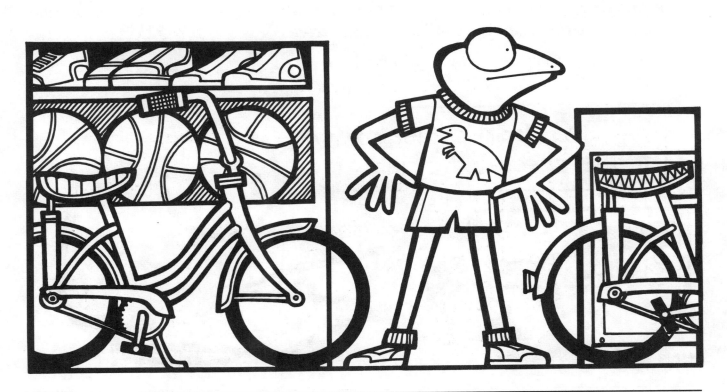

Lost in a Store

- Stay inside the store. Don't leave to look for your dad.

- Go to a cashier or to the store manager. Explain that you have become separated from your dad. Ask to have him paged.

- Say your dad's name clearly so that the person doing the paging pronounces it correctly. Wait with the cashier or store manager until your dad arrives.

- Thank the person for helping you find your dad.

Parents' Corner

When your family goes to a crowded place like a department store, supermarket, theme park, or movie theater, pick a meeting spot as soon as you get there. Then, if someone in your family accidentally gets separated, you'll know where to go to find one another.

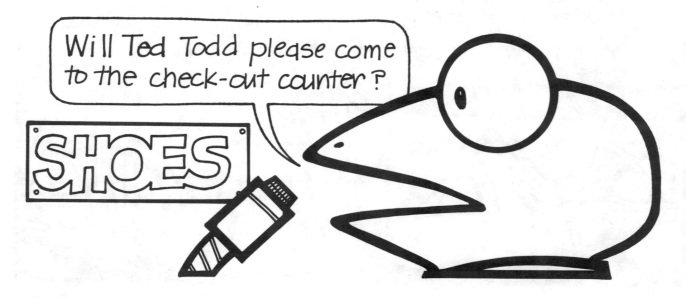

Safety Belts

You are sitting in the back seat of the car on a trip to visit your grandmother. You want to take off your safety belt because it isn't very comfortable and you want to move around in the car.

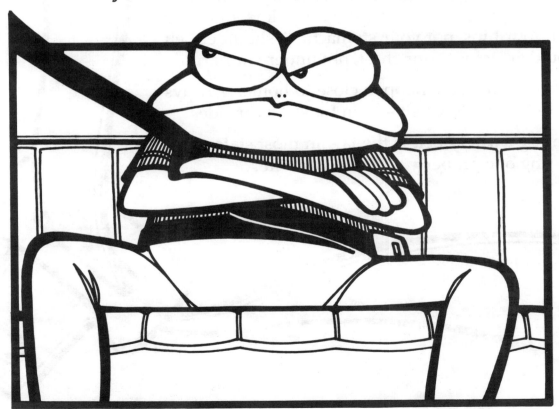

Safety Belts

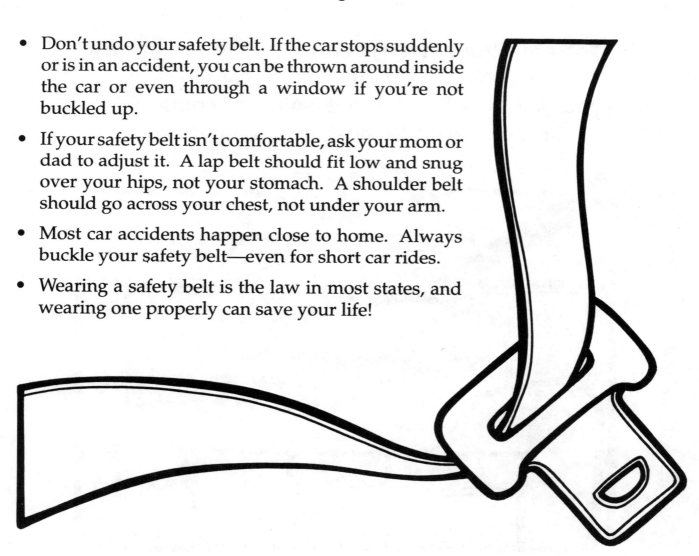

- Don't undo your safety belt. If the car stops suddenly or is in an accident, you can be thrown around inside the car or even through a window if you're not buckled up.

- If your safety belt isn't comfortable, ask your mom or dad to adjust it. A lap belt should fit low and snug over your hips, not your stomach. A shoulder belt should go across your chest, not under your arm.

- Most car accidents happen close to home. Always buckle your safety belt—even for short car rides.

- Wearing a safety belt is the law in most states, and wearing one properly can save your life!

Homesickness

You're at a friend's house to spend the night,
but being away from home doesn't seem
like such a good idea anymore.
You don't want to stay, but you feel funny
telling your friend's parents how you feel.

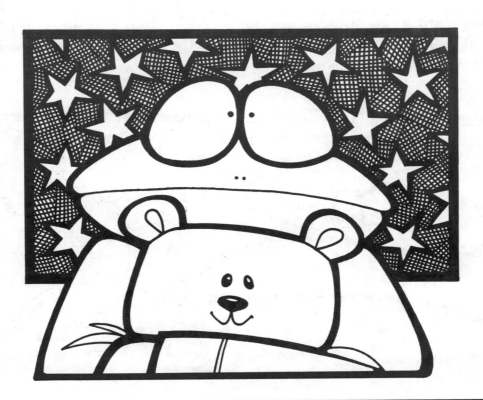

Homesickness

- Many kids feel homesick at one time or another, especially when they are sleeping away from their families for the first time.

- Don't be embarrassed about the way you feel. Tell your friend's parents. Sometimes talking about your feelings can make you feel better.

- If you still want to go home, call your mom or dad. You might feel better after you've talked to them, or they might decide to come and get you.

Safety Tip for Kids

Next time you plan to sleep away from home, bring a favorite blanket, stuffed animal, or something special with you. Familiar objects can make a strange place feel more like home.

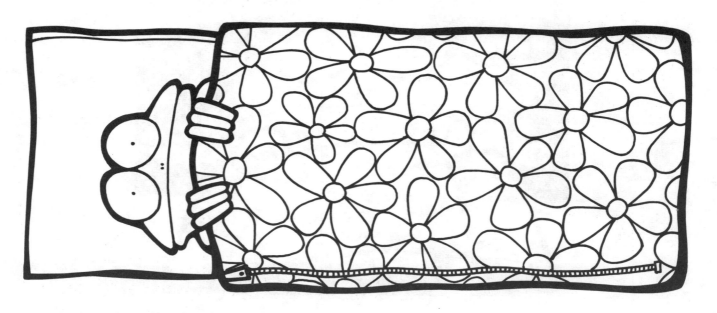

Key in the Car

You and your dad get in the car to go to the store.
Your dad realizes that he has left his wallet in the house.
He runs back to get it, leaving the car key in the ignition.

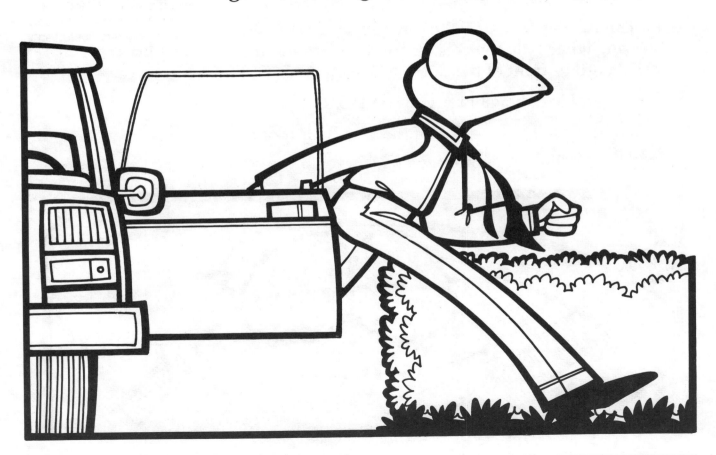

Key in the Car

- Don't touch the car key. If you accidentally start the car, it could roll. You could be badly hurt. The car might hit someone else, too, and seriously injure that person.

- Be careful not to touch the emergency brake, the steering wheel, the controls, or anything around the dashboard or front of the car.

- Sit still and calmly wait for your dad to return.

- When your dad gets back, remind him he forgot to take his car key with him.

Parents' Corner

Never leave young children alone in a car. Even when a key is not left in the ignition, a curious child can shift the car into neutral and cause it to roll.

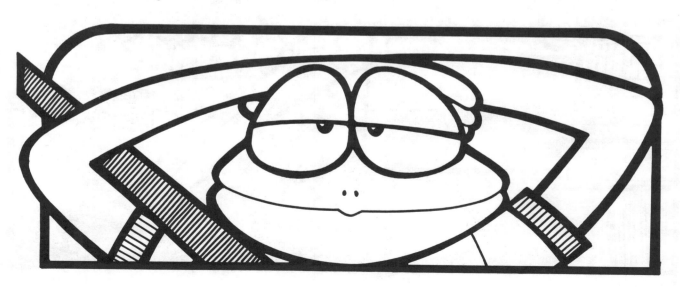

Walking on the Street

One afternoon, you are walking with your friends
to the neighborhood park for soccer practice.
Your friends begin arguing about which side
of the street to walk on. They can't agree which side
of the street is safest when there are no sidewalks.

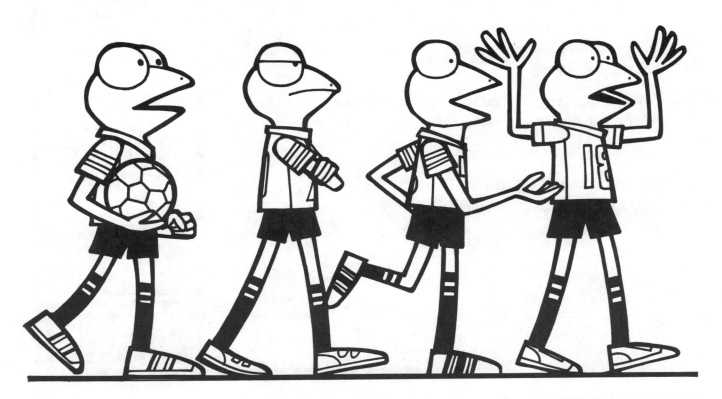

Walking on the Street

- Keep to the left and walk **facing traffic** if there are no sidewalks in your neighborhood.

- If there are sidewalks, be sure to use them.

- Cross the street only at corners, not in the middle of the block.

- Stop at the curb before crossing. Listen and look for traffic to the left, to the right, and to the left again. Wait until the street is clear and no traffic is coming before you cross.

- Pay attention and keep looking for cars until you and your friends have crossed the street safely.

- Never run into the street.

- Cross the street together. The drivers of cars can see large groups easier than one person.

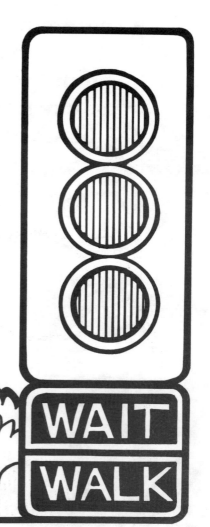

Bed-Wetting

Your family is planning a trip to your aunt and uncle's house.
You've never met this aunt and uncle or their kids,
and you're worried about staying at their house
because sometimes you wet the bed at night.

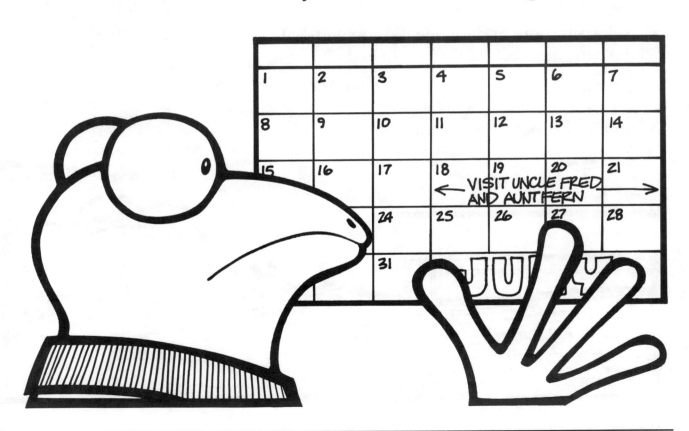

Bed-Wetting

- You aren't alone. Many kids have this problem. There are things you can do to help keep your bed dry.

- Don't drink water or other liquids after dinner.

- Go to the bathroom just before you climb into bed.

- Ask your mom or dad to wake you and walk you to the bathroom before they go to bed .

- Put a large, folded towel in your bed or sleeping bag. When you sleep away from home, have a change of underwear or pajamas handy, just in case.

Parents' Corner

A flannel-coated rubber sheet placed between the mattress pad and the bottom bed sheet will keep the mattress from getting wet and will make middle-of-the-night bed changes easier.

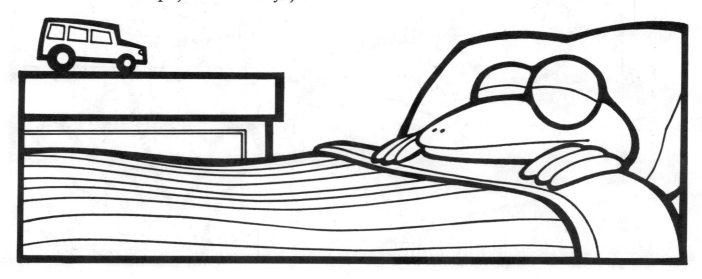

Trick-or-Treating

You have just returned home after trick-or-treating on Halloween. You dump out your bag of goodies and find several pieces of unwrapped candy.

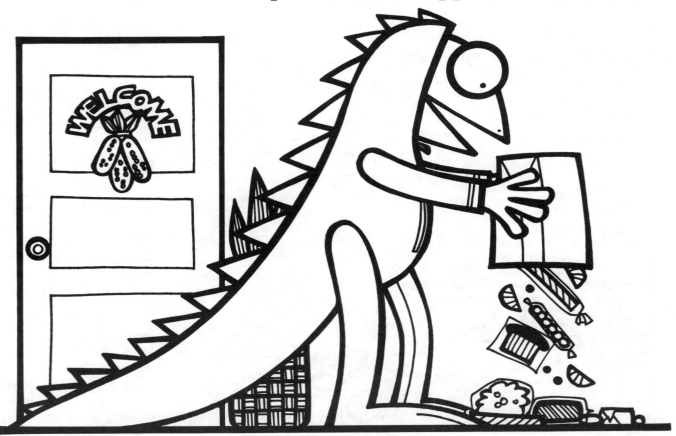

Trick-or-Treating

- When you get home, help mom or dad inspect **all** the candy and goodies you have collected.

- Throw out anything that isn't wrapped and completely sealed.

- Some hospitals will x-ray treats collected on Halloween to be sure they are safe. Ask your mom or dad to check with your local hospital to see if it has such a program.

Safety Tips for Kids

- Go trick-or-treating with friends—never by yourself. Make sure a responsible adult goes along with your group. Ask the adult in your group to carry a flashlight for you.

- Be sure your costume, or a large part of it, is a light color that can be seen at night.

- Go only to homes where the lights are on.

- Trick-or-treat in familiar neighborhoods and at the homes of friends or people you know.

- If your costume has a mask, be sure you can see clearly. After you leave each house, lift up your mask so you can see better as you walk between houses.

- When you trick-or-treat, be sure you walk—don't run, and cross the street carefully with your group.

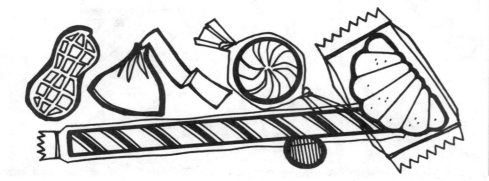

Thunderstorm

One Sunday afternoon, you are playing soccer
in the park with a group of your friends.
The sky grows dark. Rain begins to fall.
You hear loud claps of thunder
and see bolts of lightning.

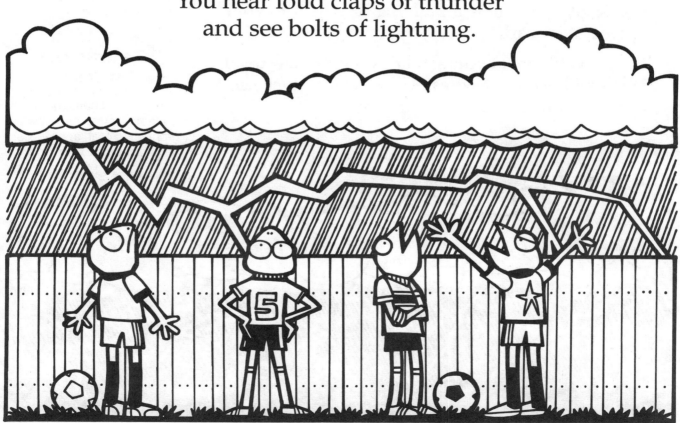

Thunderstorm

- Lightning can be very dangerous. A lightning bolt is a powerful surge of electricity. It can go from cloud to cloud, or it can hit the ground. It often strikes the highest thing in its path and can even hit people!

- If possible, get inside a building or return to your home if it is nearby.

- Keep away from anything made of metal, electrical poles, and overhead wires. These can conduct electricity toward you if you are nearby.

Parents' Corner

Make sure that all household antennas are properly grounded.

Safety Tip for Kids

If you're at home during a thunderstorm, stay away from electrical appliances, especially the television set.

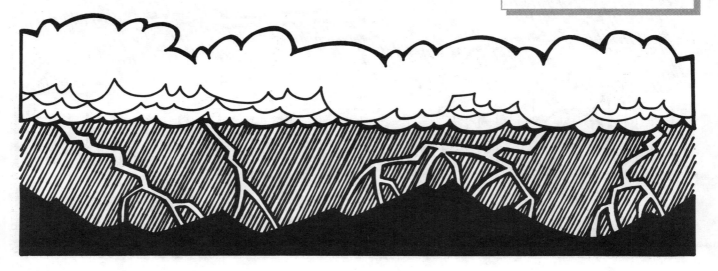

Gun in the House

When you are playing at a friend's house,
she shows you where her dad's gun is kept.
She asks if you want to see it. Then your friend
starts to take it out so the two of you can play with it.

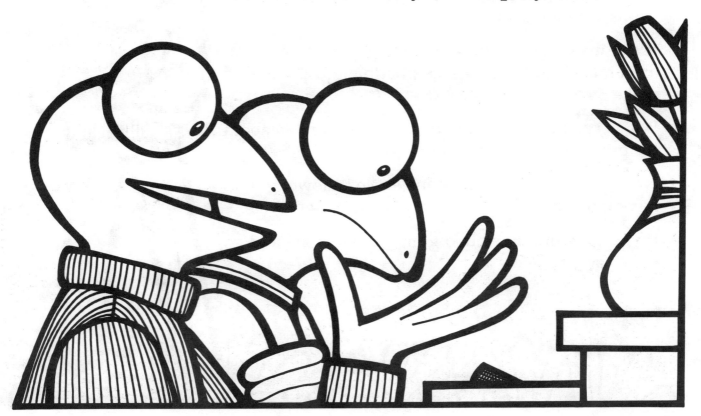

Gun in the House

- Guns are weapons, not toys. A gun can injure or kill a person.

- Leave the room right away.

- Tell her parents immediately so they can stop her from hurting herself or someone else.

- If she insists on playing with the gun and no adults are around, call 911. If it is possible, go home and make the call.

- It is very important that you tell your parents about the gun when you get home.

- Never point a gun at someone else or allow a gun to be pointed at you, even as part of a game or a joke.

- If you find an unattended gun, leave it alone and go get an adult.

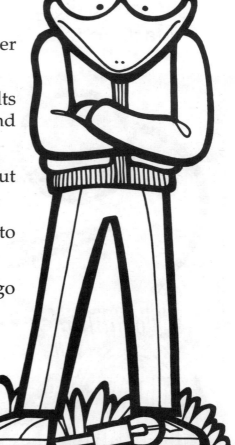

Bad Touching

You go to a movie with your older sister.
While you are sitting in the dark theater,
the man in the chair next to yours
puts his hand in your lap.

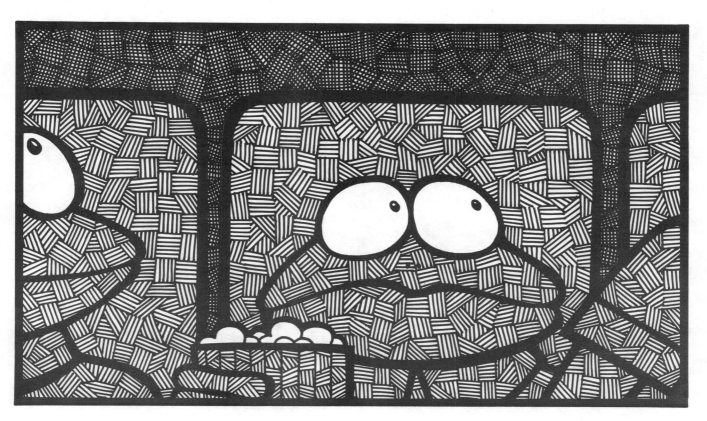

Bad Touching

- Scream for help immediately.

- Ask people around you for help.

- If no one comes to help, go with your sister to the lobby right away. Tell an usher or other theater employee what happened.

- Describe where you were sitting. If you can, describe what the stranger looked like and what he was wearing.

- Let your mom or dad know what happened.

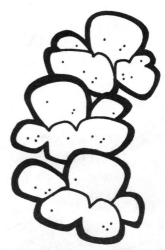

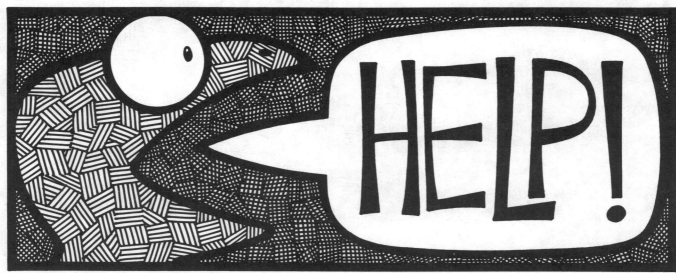

First Aid

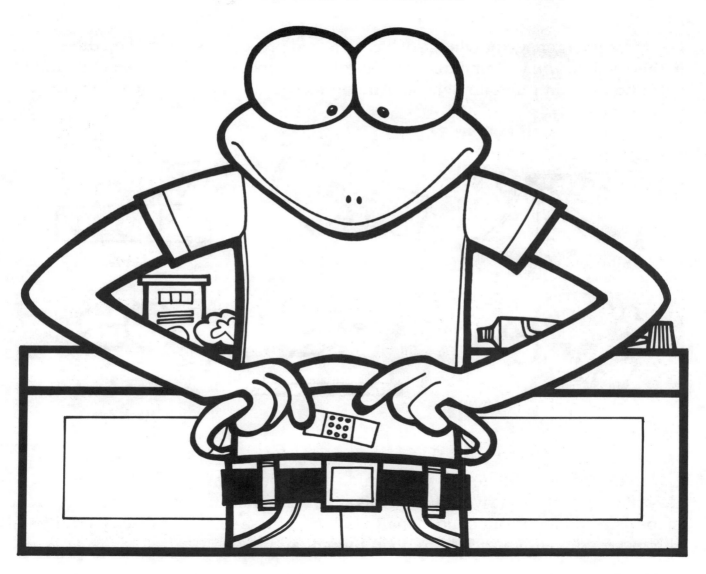

First Aid

In any emergency, knowledge of basic first aid procedures can make a difference. In this section, you will find descriptions of emergency situations your child might encounter anytime and anywhere. Among these situations are

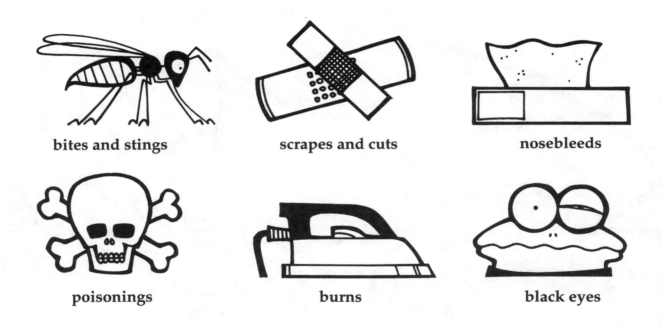

bites and stings   **scrapes and cuts**   **nosebleeds**

poisonings   **burns**   **black eyes**

First, read the situation to your child. Next, have your child think about and describe what he or she would do in this situation. Then, turn the page and read the steps listed there to your child. Finally, talk over these steps and discuss additional things you'd want your child to do in this situation.

Animal Bite

You are throwing a ball for your neighbor's dog to catch. In his excitement, he bites your hand when he tries to get the ball. Your hand starts to bleed.

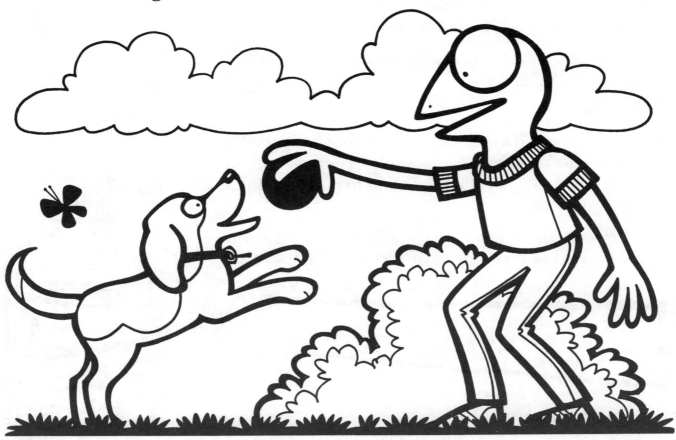

Animal Bite

- Tell your mom, dad, or another adult about the bite right away.

- Have an adult help you hold a sterile (clean) gauze pad firmly on the bite until the bleeding stops. Then wash the bite thoroughly with soap and water.

- Your mom or dad may use medicine to clean the bite.

- Ask your mom or dad to cover the area with a bandage.

- Your mom or dad should talk to your neighbor to be sure the dog has had his shots. They can get the name of the dog's vet if they want to make sure that the dog's shots are current.

- Your mom or dad should also talk to a doctor about the bite to see if you need further attention.

Safety Tip for Kids

If you are ever bitten by a stray animal, make sure that someone contacts animal control officers immediately so they can catch the animal. They will watch the animal to find out if it has rabies and will report what they learn to your doctor.

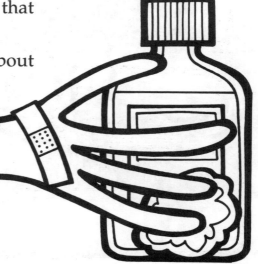

Cut Finger

While you are helping your dad
unload the dishwasher,
you cut your finger on a knife
that is sticking up in the tray.

Cut Finger

- Wrap a clean dish towel or cloth napkin snugly around your finger. Apply pressure to stop the bleeding.

- Wash the cut with soap and water.

- Ask your mom, dad, or another adult to put medicine and a bandage on the cut.

Safety Tip for Kids

When the dishwasher is loaded, be sure that knives, forks, or any kitchen utensils with sharp points are placed point **down** in the tray.

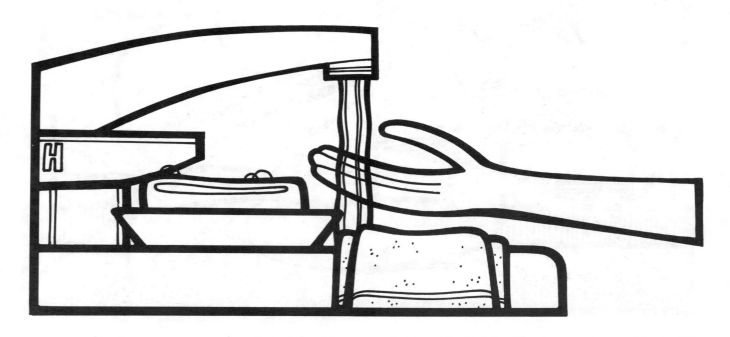

Tick Bite

While camping with your family
in a national park, you discover a tick on your leg.

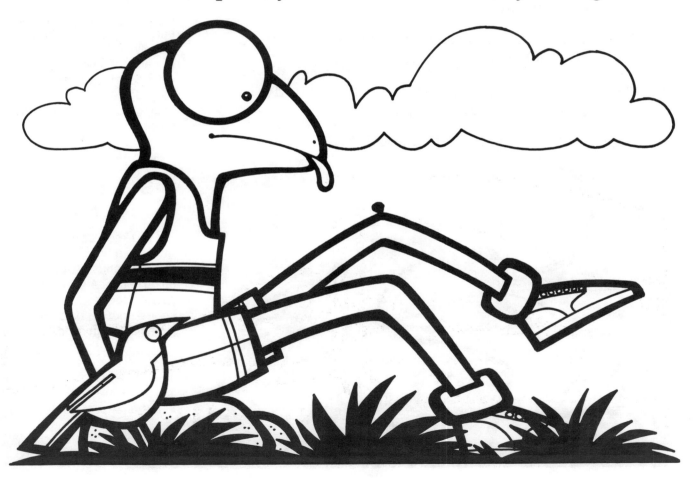

Tick Bite

- If you find a tick on your body, Mom or Dad should remove it with fine tweezers by pulling slowly with a twisting motion.

- Once the tick has been removed, wash the area around the tick bite with soap and water.

- Ask your mom or dad to apply medicine to the bite to kill the germs. Don't scratch the bite.

Parents' Corner

Ticks can carry several illnesses, including Lyme disease. Watch the bite area closely. If it becomes swollen and inflamed or if your child develops a fever, see your doctor. Ask to have your child tested for Lyme disease.

Safety Tips for Kids

If you know ticks are common in an area, wear long-sleeved shirts with snug-fitting necks. Also wear long pants, socks, and tennis shoes—not sandals. Wearing a hat is a good idea, too.

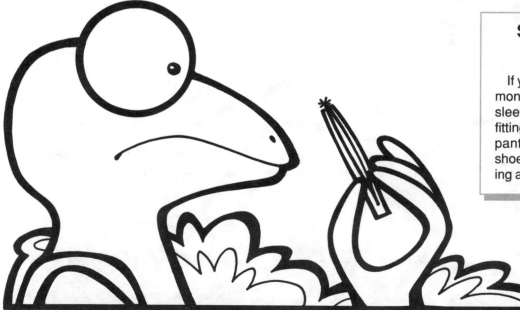

Bee Sting

When you are playing outside your house, a bee stings you on the arm. The skin around the sting turns red and begins to swell. It hurts.

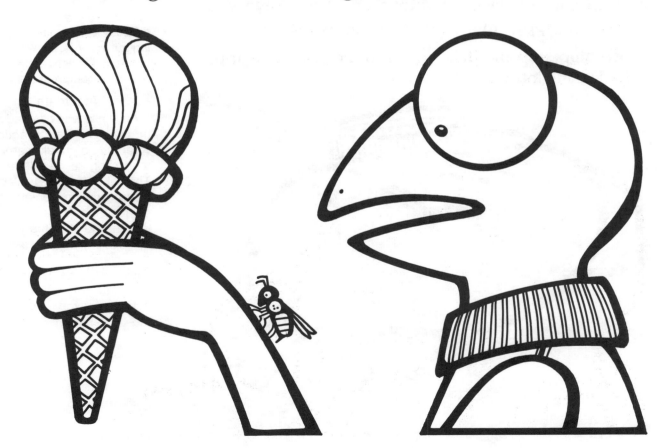

Bee Sting

- Ask Mom or Dad to remove the stinger with tweezers, being careful not to touch the end of the stinger which will push more venom into the sting.

- Run cold water over your arm. Then have your parents apply an ice pack if one is available.

- To help stop the itch, your mom or dad can apply calamine lotion.

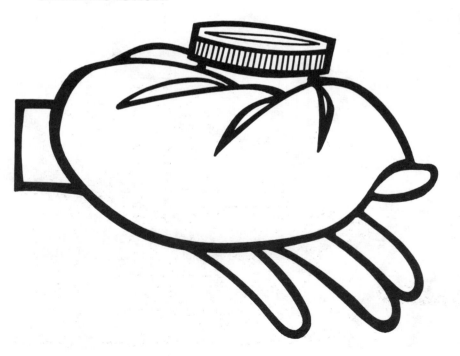

Parents' Corner

Some people have severe allergic reactions to insect bites. Some symptoms of an allergic reaction include difficulty in breathing, breaking out in hives, swelling, an increased pulse rate, and a drop in blood pressure.

What to do

Any child who has had an unusual or bad reaction when stung should carry a "bee sting kit" at all times. This kit, which is available by prescription, contains an epinephrine (adrenalin) injection and in some cases an antihistamine that can be administered orally. The child should be taken to a hospital for emergency treatment, even after the kit has been used.

Poison Oak or Ivy

In the evening, after going on a picnic with your family, you discover a rash all over your legs. Your grandmother tells you it's from poison ivy.

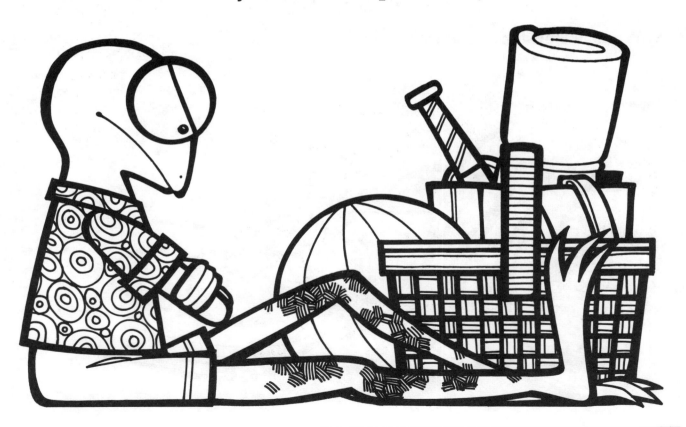

137

Poison Oak or Ivy

- Get help gently washing your legs with soap and water to remove the oil from the plant.

- Don't scrub hard with a cloth or brush.

- Ask Mom, Dad, or Grandmother to put calamine lotion on your legs to help stop the itching.

- When blisters form, don't scratch them.

Safety Tip for Kids

Learn to watch for, recognize, and stay away from poison oak or poison ivy. This is what they look like:

poison oak   poison ivy

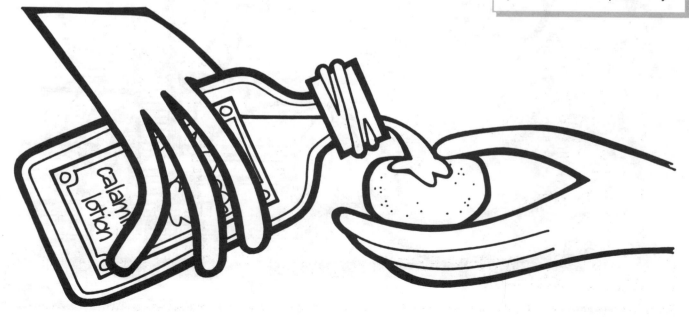

A Bad Fall

You are playing tag in your back yard.
All of a sudden, your left ankle
twists and you fall down.
Your ankle is throbbing with pain.

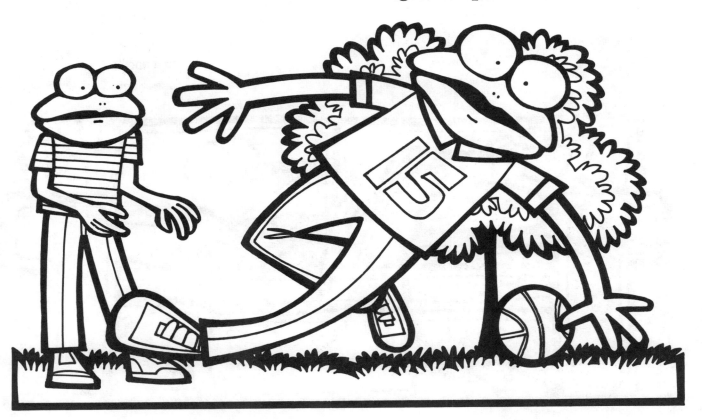

A Bad Fall

- Call for help or send a friend to find an adult.

- Have Mom or Dad put an ice pack on your ankle to make it feel better and to reduce the swelling. If it doesn't cause more pain, try to raise your ankle so that it is higher than your hips.

Parents' Corner

It's often impossible to tell the difference between a bad sprain and a break without x-rays. If your child's ankle continues to hurt even when he or she isn't putting any weight on it, a bone may be broken. Take your child to a doctor.

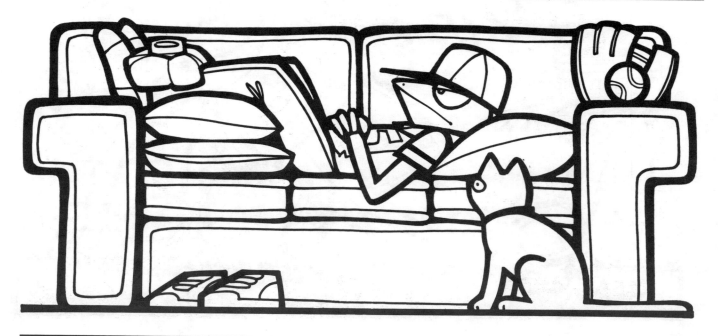

Scraped Knee

While jumping rope in front of your house, you trip, fall, and scrape your knee.

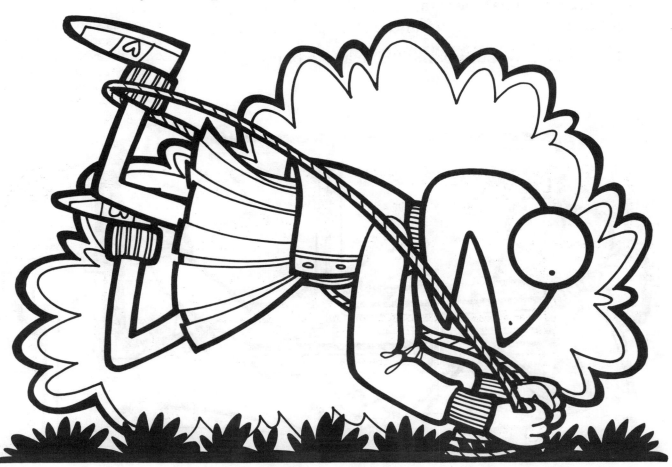

Scraped Knee

- Go inside and tell your mom or dad what happened.

- Your mom or dad will use a clean cloth to wipe away any loose dirt near the scrape, and then will wash the area with soap and water and gently pat it dry.

- Mom or Dad will apply medicine and a bandage to your knee.

Parents' Corner

When skin is broken, there is the possibility of infection. If the area around the scrape becomes hot, painful, or swollen, have your child see a doctor at once.

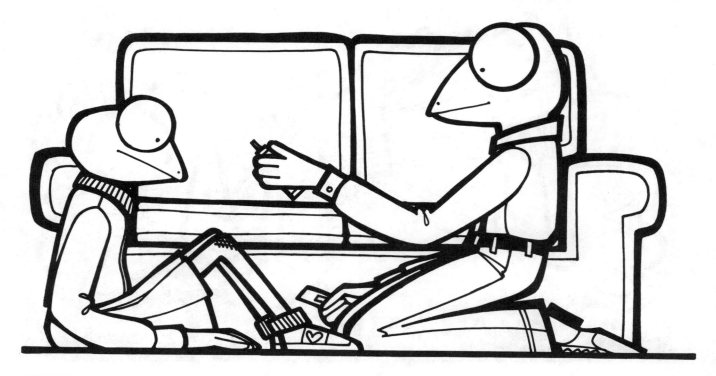

Clothes on Fire

You are camping with your family
and roasting marshmallows at the campfire.
A spark from a burning log catches your clothes on fire.

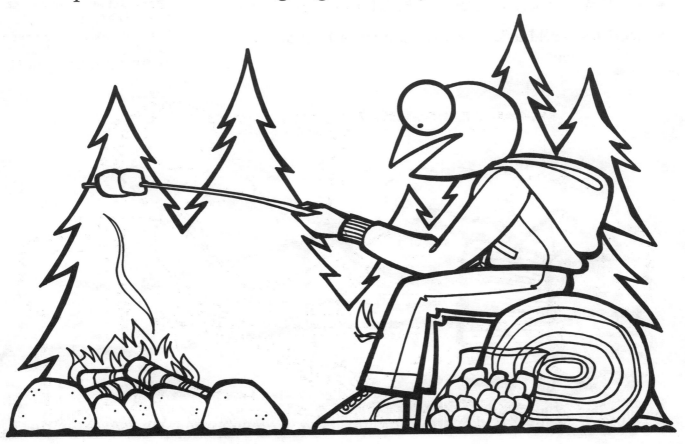

Clothes on Fire

- **STOP** – Don't run for help. Running will fan the flames and make the fire burn faster. Shout to your mom or dad for help.

- **DROP** – Drop to the ground and cover your face.

- **ROLL** – Roll back and forth to put out the flames.

Parents' Corner

Apply cool water to the burn area as soon as possible. Get emergency care for your child immediately.

Be sure your child is familiar with fire safety. Practice the STOP, DROP, and ROLL procedure.

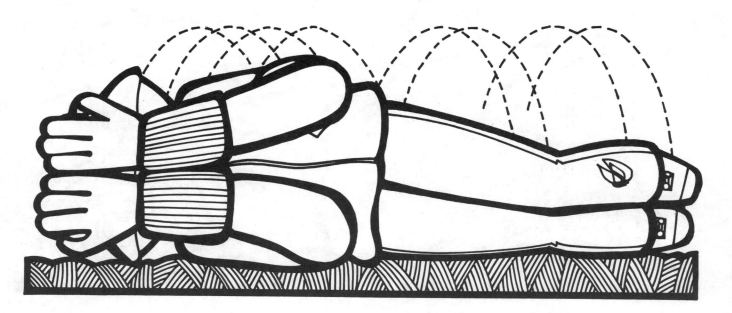

Sand in the Eye

While you are building a castle at the beach,
a little kid runs by and kicks up sand.
A piece of sand gets in your eye.

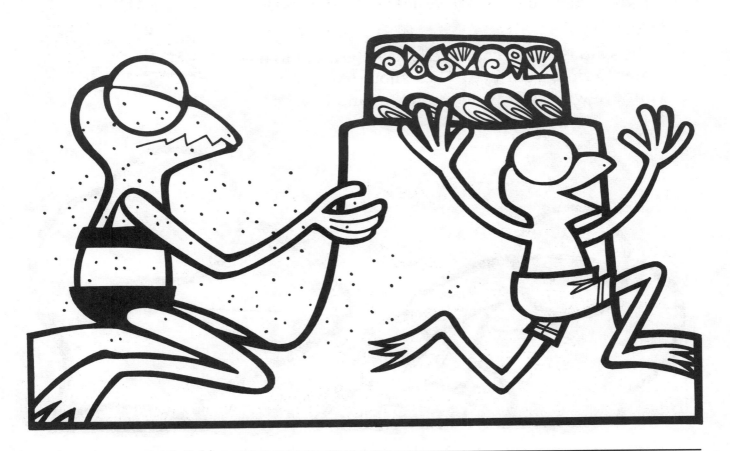

Sand in the Eye

- Don't rub your eye.

- If the sand is on your eyelid, have your mom, dad, or another adult try to remove the sand by touching it lightly with the moistened corner of a clean handkerchief or cloth.

- If the sand is under your eyelid, ask the adult to use water to rinse your eye. They should keep rinsing your eye with clear water until the sand is gone.

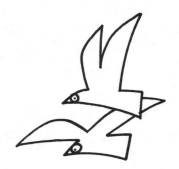

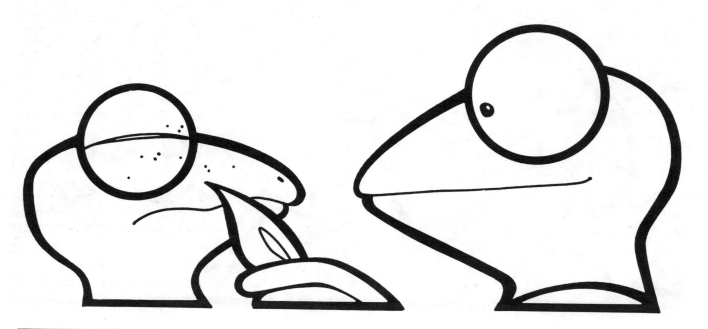

Burned Finger

Someone has left a hot iron on the counter to cool. When you are getting a snack, you accidentally touch the hot iron. It burns your finger.

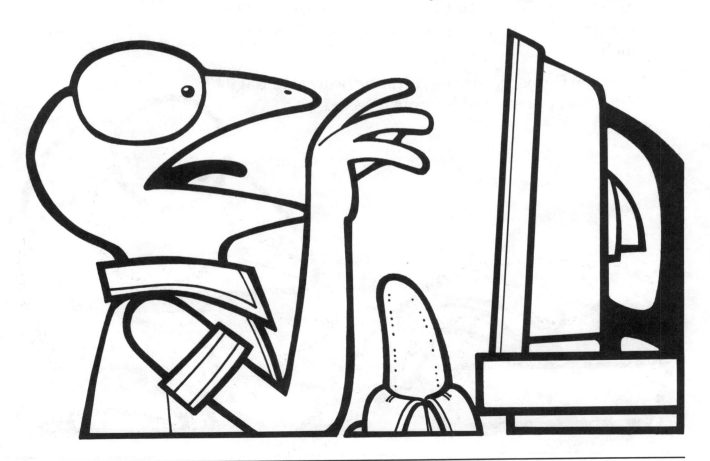

Burned Finger

- Tell your mom or dad about your finger.

- Put your burned finger in a bowl of cool water to help it feel better.

- Ask Mom or Dad to put medicine made especially for burns on your finger so the burn won't hurt as much.

- If a blister forms, protect it with an adhesive bandage so it doesn't break and become infected.

Parents' Corner

Never leave hot appliances, such as irons or frying pans, in easy reach of children.

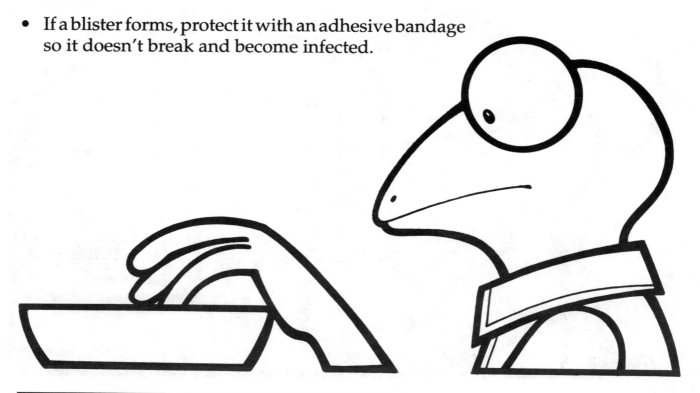

Black Eye

When you are wrestling with your older brother,
he accidentally hits you above your eye with his elbow.
The area above your eye gets red and puffy. Before long,
the skin around your eye begins to turn black and blue.

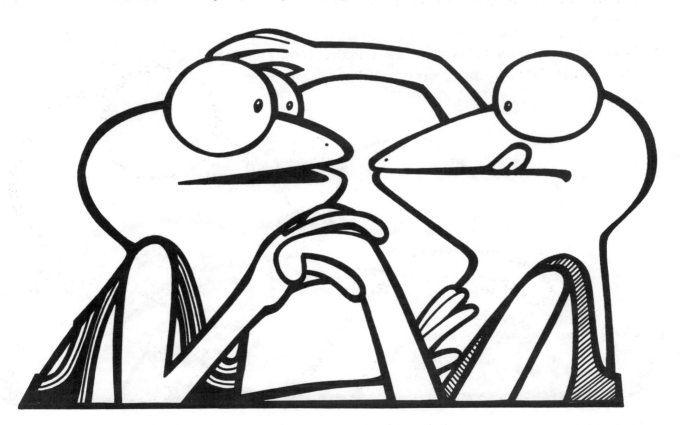

Black Eye

- Don't rub or wash your eye.

- Cover your uninjured eye with your hand and make sure you can still see clearly with the eye that was hit.

- Your mom or dad should check to make sure that you aren't hurt anywhere else.

- To ease the pain and slow the swelling, hold an ice pack over your eye. You can also soak a small towel in ice water, wring it out, and hold it on the bruised area around your eye.

Parents' Corner

A black eye actually is a bruise. Discoloration is caused by the breaking of tiny blood vessels around the eye. Your child doesn't need medical attention for a black eye unless the skin has been cut, the eye itself has been injured, or facial bones have been broken.

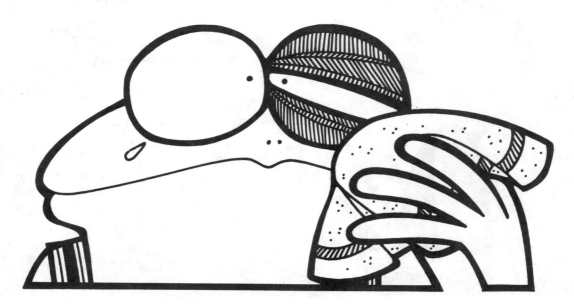

Nosebleed

While you are playing ball with your sister, you get hit in the face. Your nose starts to bleed.

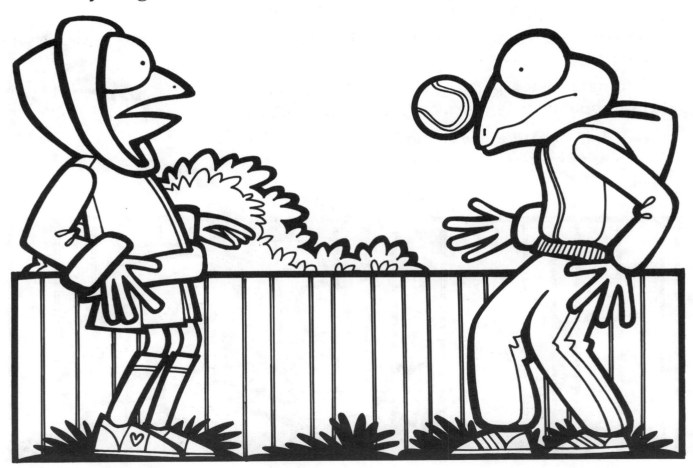

Nosebleed

- Ask your sister to get your mom or dad right away.

- While she goes for help, sit down and lean forward. Pinch the soft part of your nose together. Stay in this position for 5 to 10 minutes, or until the bleeding stops.

- Holding a folded piece of wet paper towel under your upper lip may also help slow the bleeding.

- Ask Mom or Dad to lay a cold, damp washcloth or towel across your face to help you feel more comfortable.

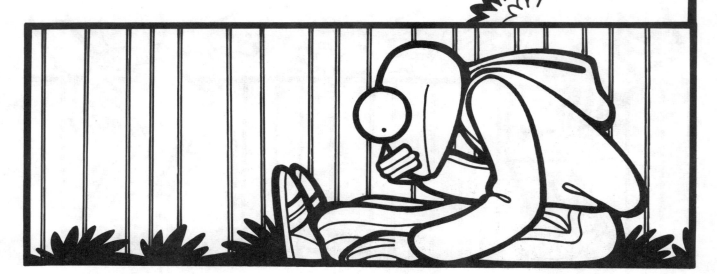

Tooth Knocked Out

When you're riding your bike, you hit a loose rock
and lose your balance. You fall forward and hit
your mouth on the handlebars. Your mouth
is bleeding, and you discover that one of
your front teeth is missing.

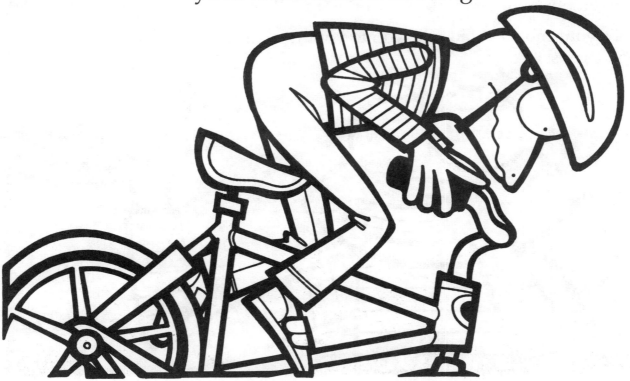

Tooth Knocked Out

- Tell your mom or dad right away.

- Find your missing tooth and gently rinse it in cool water. Don't use soap or detergent. Don't scrub the tooth with a brush or cloth.

- With help from your mom or dad, carefully place the rinsed tooth back into its socket and hold it there.

- Have your mom or dad take you to your dentist as soon as possible.

Safety Tip for Kids

If it isn't possible to keep your tooth in its socket, put it in a glass of cool milk or water. Don't forget to take it with you when you go to the dentist!

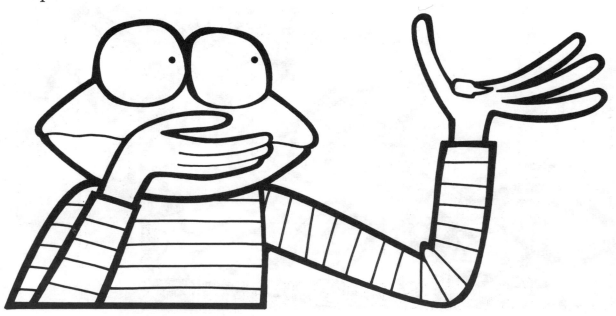

Injured Back

Your mom trips and falls on the stairs.
She says that her back and neck hurt.
You are the only person there to help her.

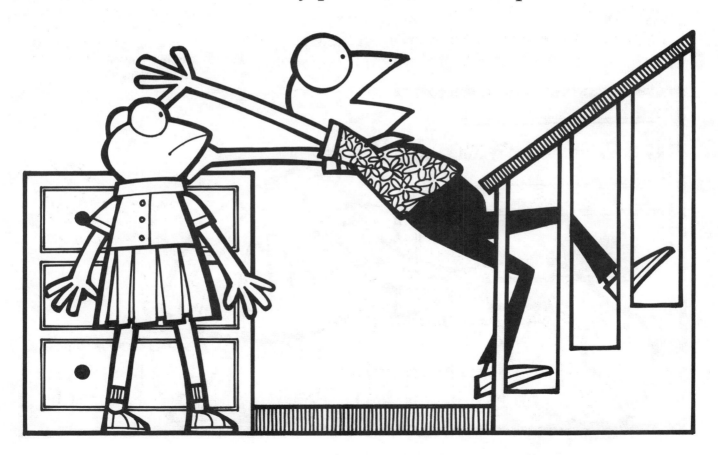

Injured Back

- Tell your mom to lie flat. Don't let her try to get up.

- Dial 911. Tell the operator what has happened and give your name and address.

- Ask your mom if she wants you to cover her with a blanket. Let her know that help is on the way.

Safety Tip for Kids

Whenever you make a phone call in an emergency, be sure to say your name and address slowly and clearly. You want the operator to understand you easily.

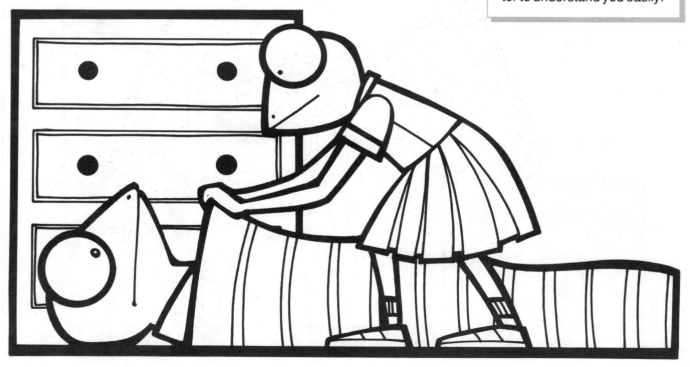

Just for Fun
Kids' Activities

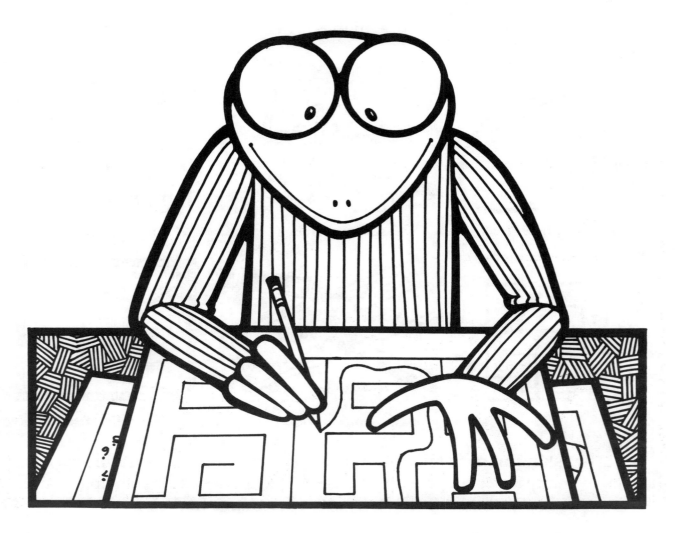

Just for Fun
Kids' Activities

In this section, you will find fun activities to help you become safety smart. These activities include

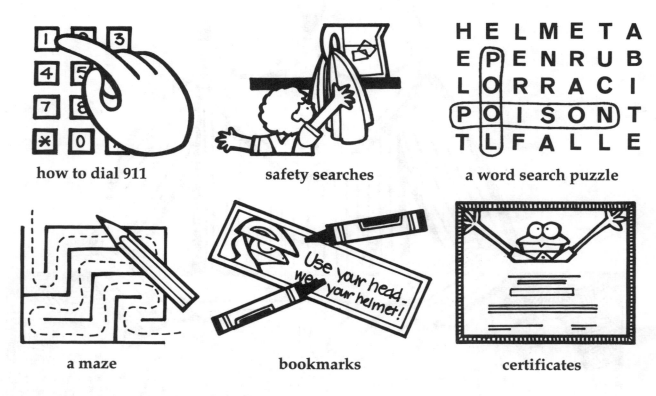

how to dial 911   safety searches   a word search puzzle

a maze   bookmarks   certificates

Begin by asking mom or dad to help you select activities that you will enjoy. Have them go over any instructions with you. Be sure to ask an adult for help if you need assistance with any of these projects or activities. Have fun!

How to Dial 911

Here's what to do when you need to dial 911.

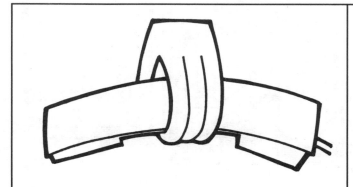

1. Pick up the telephone receiver.

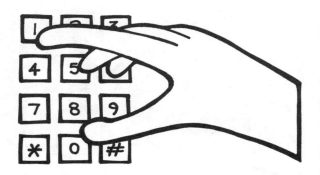

2. Dial 911. First press **9**, then **1**, then another **1**.

407 River Drive

3. When the operator answers, he or she will ask you for:
   - the telephone number you are calling from
   - your first and last name
   - your address
   - a description of the problem

   Be sure to speak slowly and clearly.

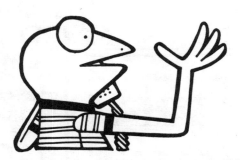

4. Stay on the phone with the operator until he or she tells you to hang up.

If you are away from home and have to dial 911, use a pay phone. You **don't** have to put any money in the pay phone to dial 911. Follow the steps listed above.

Kitchen Safety Search

Find the safety hazards in this picture.

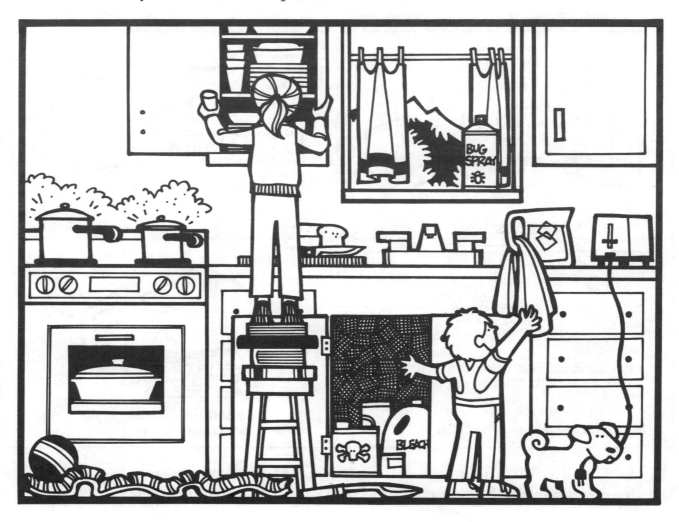

Safety Code

The message on the next page is written in this code.
To read it, write the letters on the lines.

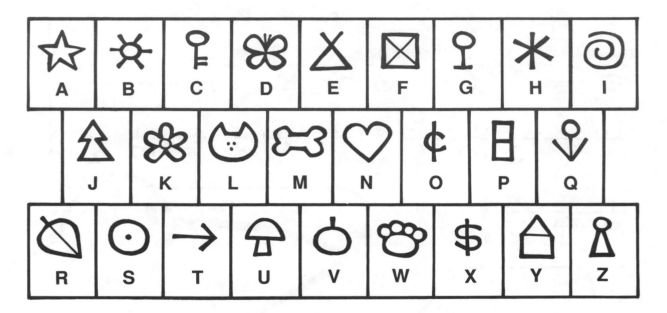

Now use the code to write secret messages to your friends.

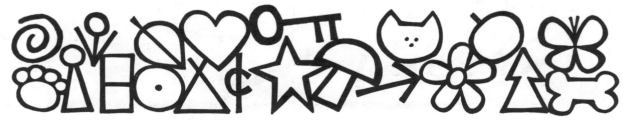

Crack the Code

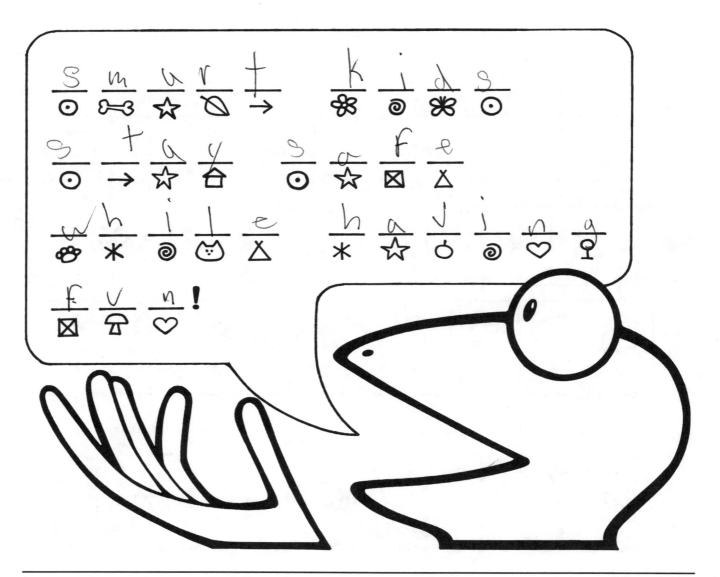

Safety Bookmarks

Photocopy and color the bookmarks on these two pages. Then cut them out and mount them on strips of colored paper. Share the bookmarks that you make with your family and friends.

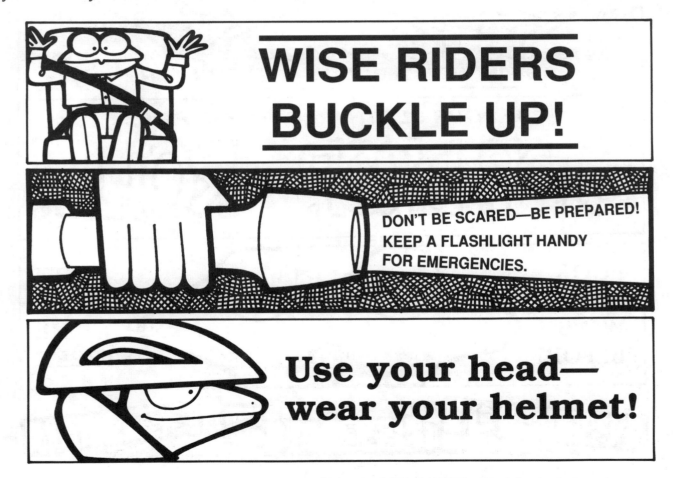

Safety Bookmarks
(continued)

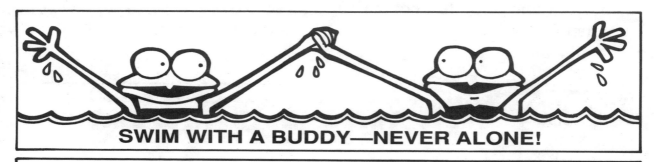

SWIM WITH A BUDDY—NEVER ALONE!

IF YOUR CLOTHING CATCHES FIRE,

STOP, DROP AND ROLL!

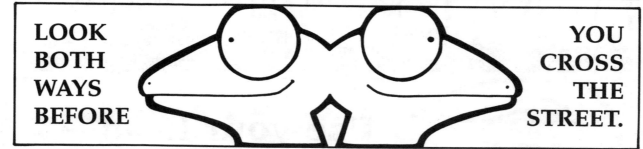

LOOK BOTH WAYS BEFORE YOU CROSS THE STREET.

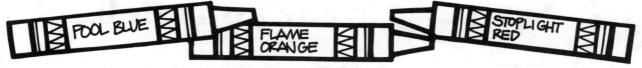

POOL BLUE   FLAME ORANGE   STOPLIGHT RED

Safety Certificates

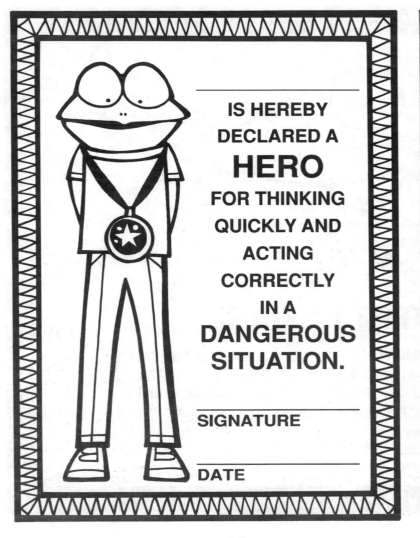

_____

IS HEREBY
DECLARED A
HERO
FOR THINKING
QUICKLY AND
ACTING
CORRECTLY
IN A
**DANGEROUS
SITUATION.**

_____
SIGNATURE

_____
DATE

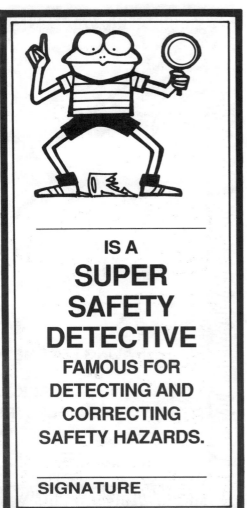

_____

IS A
**SUPER
SAFETY
DETECTIVE**
FAMOUS FOR
DETECTING AND
CORRECTING
SAFETY HAZARDS.

_____
SIGNATURE

Safety Certificates
(continued)

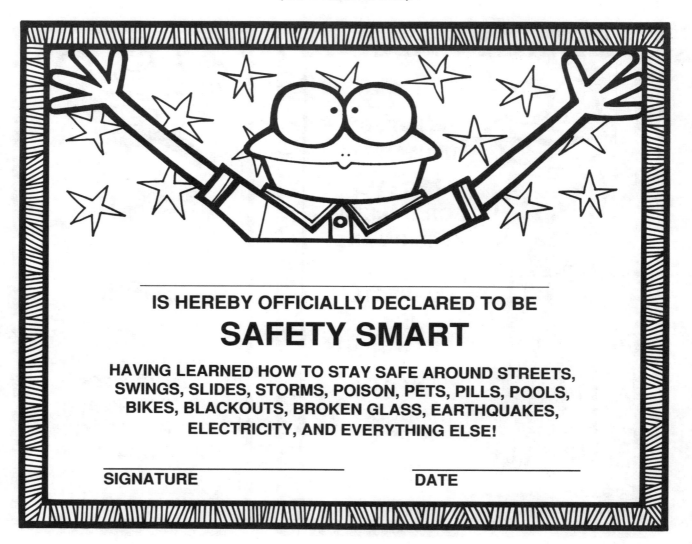

IS HEREBY OFFICIALLY DECLARED TO BE

SAFETY SMART

HAVING LEARNED HOW TO STAY SAFE AROUND STREETS, SWINGS, SLIDES, STORMS, POISON, PETS, PILLS, POOLS, BIKES, BLACKOUTS, BROKEN GLASS, EARTHQUAKES, ELECTRICITY, AND EVERYTHING ELSE!

SIGNATURE

DATE

Answer Key

Kitchen Safety Search
Page 162
Here are some of the hazards. You may have found additional hazards in this picture and the ones on page 163 and 164.

    spoon and ball on floor
    loose rug
    puppy playing with electrical cord
    toddler reaching for pitcher with a towel through the handle
    child balancing on books and stool
    knife left out on counter
    bug spray in food preparation area
    overhanging pot handles on stove
    poisons in cupboard under sink

Bathroom Safety Search
Page 163
young child unattended in the bathtub
bottle of pills left out
loose area rug
soap left on edge of bathtub
medicine cabinet door left open
electric rollers plugged in and left unattended
cleaning fluids left out on counter
toilet lid left open
dangling hair dryer
toy on floor

Outdoor Safety Search
Page 164
children on bicycle not wearing helmets and riding double
ball and bat on sidewalk
loose dog (no collar or tags)
rake on lawn
hose across walkway
skates on steps
toddler alone in pool
hot barbecue
child running with stick
kite being flown near power lines
broken window

Safety Dot-to-Dot
Page 165

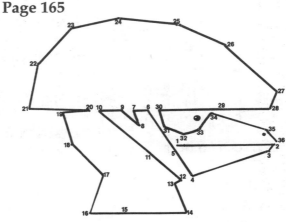

Answer Key
(continued)

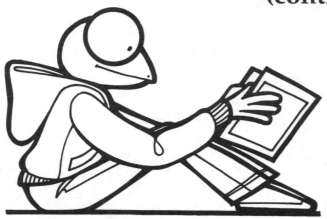

Safety Maze
Page 169

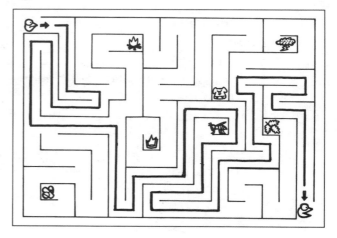

Safety Word Search Puzzle
Page 166

Crack the Code
Page 168

SMART KIDS STAY SAFE
WHILE HAVING FUN!

Calling 911!
Page 170

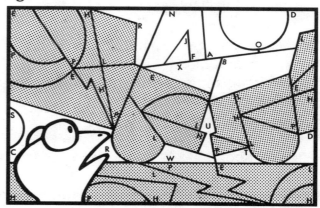

Pages for Parents
Lists, Checklists, and How-To Information

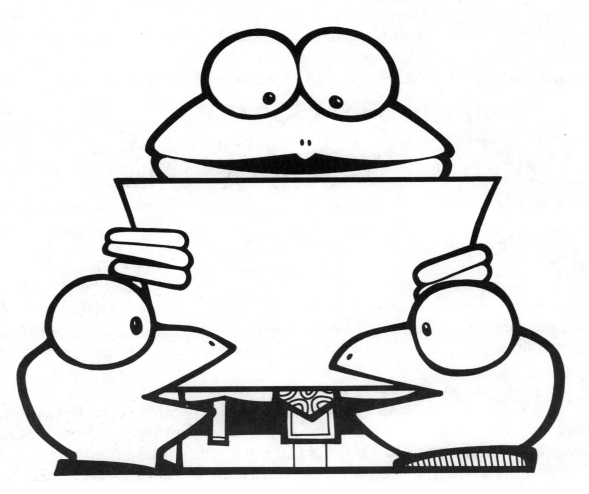

Pages for Parents
Lists, Checklists, and How-To Information

In this section, you will find a collection of practical lists and checklists to help you and your child prepare for minor emergencies and to avoid major ones. You'll also find practical how-to information for what to do in those unexpected situations that can involve young children. Some of the lists, checklists, and information include:

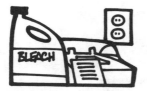

a home safety checklist

a poisonous plant checklist

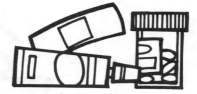

a list of first aid supplies

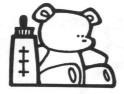

**information for
your baby-sitter**

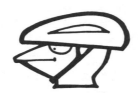

**tips on buying
a child's bike helmet**

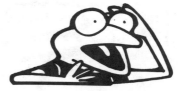

**information on helping
a choking person**

Ask your child to go through your home with you, using the checklists. Make plans to correct safety defects you find. Place the lists, such as the emergency telephone numbers and the emergency equipment and supplies, where they can be easily seen and conveniently used. Refer to them often. Update or adapt them in any way that will make them more useful for your family.

Home Safety Checklist

☐ Post emergency telephone numbers within easy view of each telephone.

☐ Install smoke alarms on each floor of your house and in all sleeping areas.

☐ Test smoke alarms once a year to be certain that they are in good working order.

☐ Replace frayed wires and defective electrical sockets.

☐ Put safety covers on electrical outlets that are not in use.

☐ Replace all burned-out light bulbs so kids don't trip and fall in dark hallways or rooms.

☐ Store potentially poisonous substances beyond the reach of small children and pets.

☐ If there are small children in the house, use safety gates to block access to stairwells.

☐ Repair or replace hall and area rugs that slip and slide.

Kitchen Safety Checklist

☐ Keep a sturdy ladder handy to help you reach objects in high places.

☐ Turn the pots and pans on your stove so that the handles point toward the back and your child can't grab them.

☐ Wipe up floor spills immediately to prevent falls in the kitchen.

☐ Store knives in a rack instead of keeping them loose in a kitchen drawer.

☐ Install a smoke detector in your kitchen. Replace the batteries yearly.

☐ Keep a fire extinguisher in the kitchen. Be sure you know how to use it in case of a kitchen fire. Check the expiration date periodically.

☐ Replace frayed electrical cords on appliances.

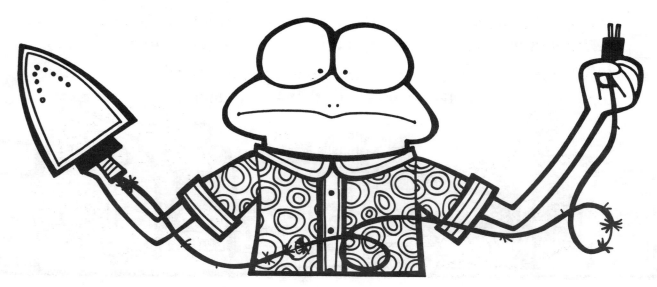

Bathroom Safety Checklist

- [ ] Store medicines beyond the reach of small children. If necessary, place a lock on your medicine cabinet to prevent your child from opening it.
- [ ] Buy medicines in child-resistant packages.
- [ ] Never use electrical appliances around water.
- [ ] Keep bathroom cleaning products such as drain and toilet cleaners in a locked cabinet out of your child's reach.
- [ ] Use nonskid rugs in the bathroom to help prevent falls.
- [ ] Use rubber mats in the bathtub and shower so your child doesn't slip.
- [ ] Keep toilet seats and lids down. Install seat locks if necessary.
- [ ] Set your hot water heater at 115° F so that your child isn't scalded in the bathtub or shower.
- [ ] Never leave a young child unattended in a bathtub, even for a minute.

Outdoor Safety Checklist

☐ Check to make sure your child is out of the area when a lawn mower or other motorized tool is being used.

☐ If you have a swimming pool, protect your child and others from accidentally drowning by installing a fence and a gate that closes automatically. Be sure the gate is locked when the pool is not in use.

☐ Enroll the adults in your family in CPR classes and your children in swimming lessons.

☐ Supervise children in your pool or spa at all times. Don't leave a young child unattended—even for a few minutes. If you have to go inside, make sure all children are out of the pool area.

☐ Pick up garden tools and put them away after they are used so your child doesn't trip on them or play with them.

☐ Have your child wear a bike helmet every time he or she rides a bike.

☐ Be sure your child is in a car seat or buckled up securely every time he or she rides in a car, even for short distances.

Poisonous Plants

Here is a partial list of common toxic plants. Some of these plants are poisonous if chewed or swallowed. Others cause rashes and other allergic reactions. Some plants are toxic to children at all times, while others are harmful only when eaten or chewed at certain stages of the plant's growth.

PLANT	POISONOUS PART(S)
aminta	all parts
azalea	all parts
bird of paradise	fruits and seeds
boxwood	all parts
buttercup	all parts
daffodil	bulb
English holly	berries
English ivy	all parts
foxglove	all parts
holly	berries
horse chestnut	all parts
iris	root
larkspur	all parts
lily-of-the-valley	all parts
mistletoe	all parts
morning glory	seeds
oleander	all parts
philodendron	all parts
poinsettia	all parts
tomato	leaves
wisteria	seeds and pod

Parent's Corner

Here are some safety tips about poisonous plants:

- Teach your child not to eat or chew **any** part of a plant he or she doesn't know is safe.
- Warn your child never to eat mushrooms found growing wild.
- Seek emergency medical treatment for your child if he or she chews or swallows a poisonous plant.
- When seeking emergency treatment, bring along part of the plant or be able to identify it.

First Aid Supply Checklist

☐ adhesive bandages in assorted sizes and shapes

☐ roll of adhesive tape

☐ sterile gauze pads

☐ roll of gauze

☐ antiseptic cream for treatment of minor cuts and scrapes

☐ first aid cream or topical anesthetic for relief of itching and pain

☐ antibacterial soap

☐ baking soda

☐ calamine lotion

☐ flashlight with batteries

☐ ipecac syrup*

☐ triangular bandages

☐ hot water bottle

☐ ice bag or ice pack

☐ children's medications

☐ pair of scissors

☐ pair of tweezers

☐ thermometer

☐ medicine (eye) dropper

☐ teaspoon for measuring

☐ rubbing alcohol

☐ plastic bags

☐ blanket

☐ disposable gloves

* Ipecac syrup is used to induce vomiting in the event of accidental poisoning.
(Call your physician or poison control center before administering ipecac.)

"I Can Do" Checklist

Instructions: Photocopy this page so that you'll be able to create a customized "I Can Do" checklist for each school-age child in your family. The responsibility you allow each child to take will vary with his or her age and maturity.

At home, I'm allowed to

YES NO

- use the toaster
- use the microwave oven
- use the stove
- use the electric can opener
- use the family computer
- turn on the radio/stereo

Use these other appliances:

_____

_____

_____

I'm allowed to

YES NO

- ride my bike to a neighbor's house
- play at a friend's house
- cross the street
- fix a sandwich using a sharp knife

Other things I'm allowed to do:

_____

_____

_____

Emergency Telephone Numbers

Instructions: Photocopy this page and fill in names and/or telephone numbers. Then photocopy the completed page so you will have enough copies to place one near each telephone. Don't forget to update the list whenever necessary.

911 or local emergency number _____

Fire department _____

Police or sheriff's department _____

Poison center _____

Family doctor _____

Mother at work _____

Father at work _____

Grandparent or other relative _____

Neighbor _____

Close friend _____

Gas company _____

Electric power company _____

Plumber _____

Electrician _____

Veterinarian _____

Other:_____ _____

Important Information for Our Baby-Sitter

Our children's names, ages, and bedtimes are

name _Briana Smith_   age _9_   bedtime _10:30_ school days

name _____   age _____   bedtime _____

name _____   age _____   bedtime _____

Our home address is _____

The nearest cross streets are _____

_____

Our home telephone number is _____

We expect to be home around _____

We can be reached at _____

If we can't be reached, you can call

    name _____   phone _____

Our doctor is

    name _____   phone _____

A relative you can call is

    name _____   phone _____

Special instructions: _____

_____

Emergency Equipment and Supplies

- [ ] batteries
- [ ] blankets
- [ ] candles
- [ ] can opener, manual
- [ ] fire extinguisher
- [ ] first aid supplies (see list on page 184)
- [ ] flashlight
- [ ] food, canned or dehydrated to last for several days

- [ ] gloves, heavy
- [ ] knife, pocket
- [ ] lantern, propane
- [ ] matches
- [ ] radio, battery- or transistor-operated
- [ ] tools—axe, broom, hammer, screwdriver, and shovel
- [ ] watch or clock
- [ ] water, bottled
- [ ] wrench, crescent

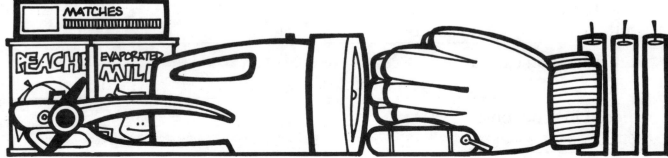

Fire Escape Routes

Would your child know how to get out of your house or apartment in case of a fire? Don't wait for an emergency. Plan fire escape routes for your family now!

Here's what to do:

- Plan **two** ways to get out of every room of your home. For example, if a doorway is blocked by fire, plan an escape route out a window. Hold practice fire drills in your home on a regular basis.

- Agree on a place outside your home where everyone will meet. This meeting place could be across the street, by your mailbox, or in front of your neighbor's house. Make sure your meeting place is in view of the front of your house.

- Decide who will be responsible for each young child in your family.

- Discuss this plan as a family. Be sure your children understand that once they have left a burning building, they should never go back inside to look for another family member. Your children should go to the designated meeting spot. If someone is missing, a fire fighter will go in and look for the person.

- Have fire drills in your house or apartment. Plan to have at least one fire drill at night, since that's when many deadly fires occur.

- If you live in a high-rise apartment, warn children not to use the elevator if there is a fire. Always use the stairs or fire escapes, or wait for the fire department if these routes are blocked.

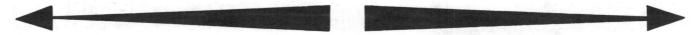

First Aid Procedures

HOW TO CHECK FOR A HEARTBEAT

Place your index and middle fingers on the side of the person's neck, as shown. Start at the Adam's apple and slide fingers to one side.

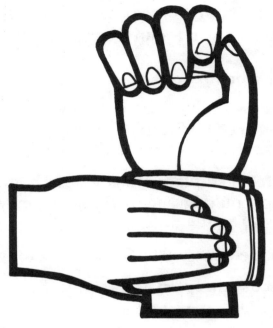

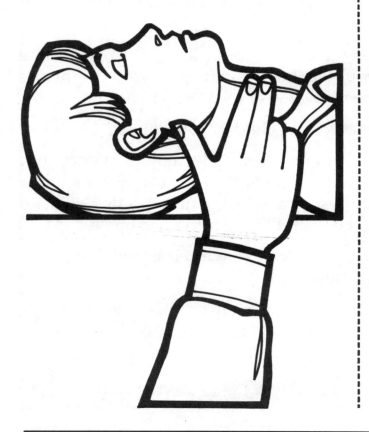

HOW TO STOP BLEEDING

- Hold a sterile gauze pad or clean, folded handkerchief on the wound.

- Apply firm, steady, direct pressure for 5 to 15 minutes.

- If the bleeding doesn't stop, or is severe, call 911 or your local emergency service.

First Aid Procedures
(continued)

HOW TO HELP A PERSON WHO IS CHOKING

Instructions: Teach your child to point to his or her throat if he or she is choking and can't talk. This is a signal to start the procedure described below.

- Call 911 or your local emergency service.

- Place your fist just above the choking person's belly button.

- Cover your fist with your other hand.

- By pulling on your fist with your other hand, apply quick thrusts of pressure between the choking person's belly button and rib cage until the object is cleared.

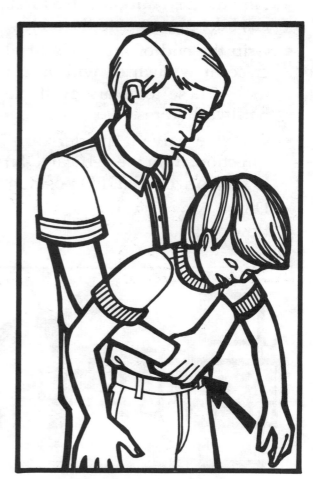

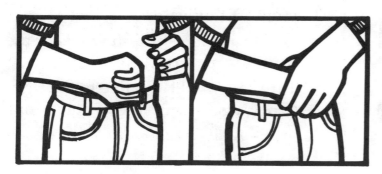

Safety Procedures

HOW TO TURN OFF THE GAS AND WATER

To shut off the gas:

- Find the gas shut-off valve located on the gas inlet pipe next to the meter.
- Grip the end of the valve firmly with a crescent wrench or with a gas shut-off tool. These tools are available at most hardware stores.
- Give the valve a quarter turn in either direction, from the vertical (ON) position to the horizontal (OFF) position.
- Doing this closes the pipe and stops the flow of gas.

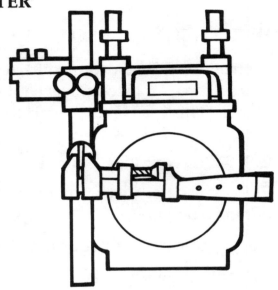

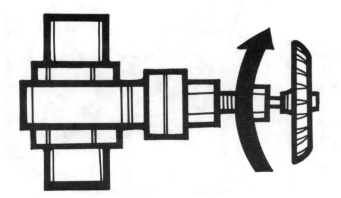

To shut off the water:

- Locate a water shut-off wheel or the main water valve.
- Turn this wheel or valve to the right (clockwise) until the water stops flowing.

Buying a Bike Helmet

Instructions: Read this page with your child
before taking your child to purchase a bike helmet.

A bicycle helmet won't keep you from falling off a bike, but it can protect your head from a bad bump. Always wear your bike helmet whenever you ride a bike.

Bike helmets come in many styles and colors. Here are some tips for finding the best one for you.

- Always try a helmet on before buying it. It should be comfortable and snug, but not too tight.

- Fasten the helmet strap. The helmet should sit level on the top of your head. It should not slide from side to side or back and forth. If you can pull the helmet off with the strap hooked, the helmet is too big.

- Wear the helmet around the store for 5 or 10 minutes. Make sure it still feels comfortable after you wear it for a while.

- The straps on most bike helmets can be adjusted for a good fit. Practice buckling and unbuckling your strap until you can do it easily. Always be sure to buckle the strap whenever you ride a bike.

- Many helmets come with foam pads in different sizes. Try using different pads to get a good, snug fit.

- Keep your helmet clean by washing it with a gentle soap and warm water.

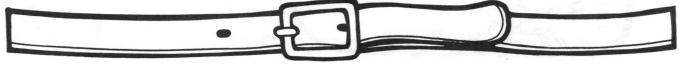

Index

Index
(continued)

Index
(continued)

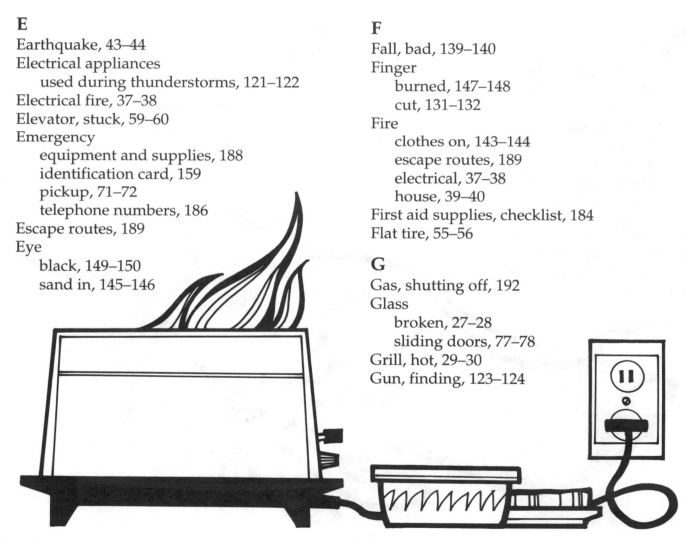

Index
(continued)

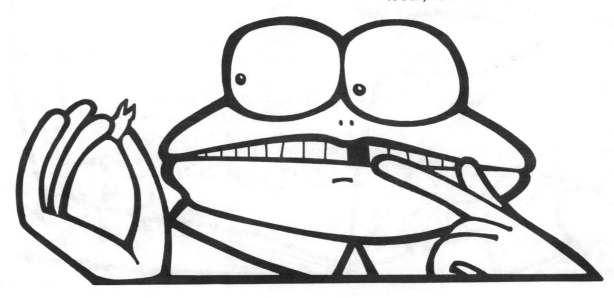

Index
(continued)

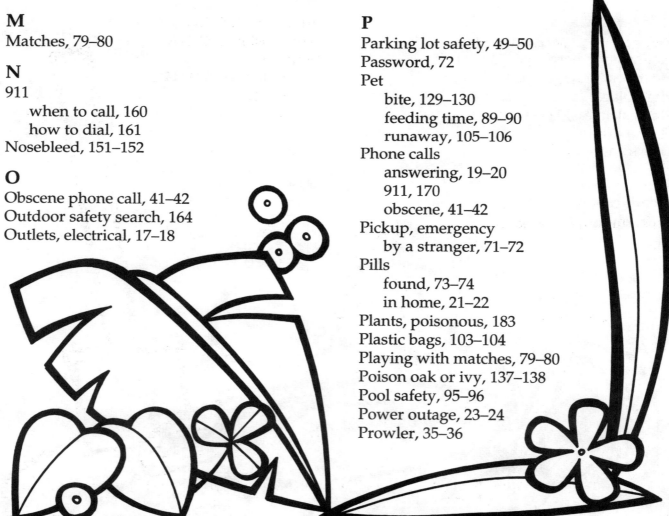

Index
(continued)

R

Refrigerator, discarded, 87–88

S

Safety belts, 109–110
Safety helmet, 51–52, 193
Sand in the eye, 145–146
Scraped knee, 141–142
Shut-off valves, gas or water, 192
Slide safety, 85–86
Stairs, playing on, 91–92
Stick, running with, 65–66

Sting, bee, 135–136
Store, lost in, 107–108
Stranger
    fondled by, 125–126
    offering ride, 71–72
Street
    chasing ball, 99–100
    crossing, 69–70
    walking on, 115–116
Swing safety, 93–94

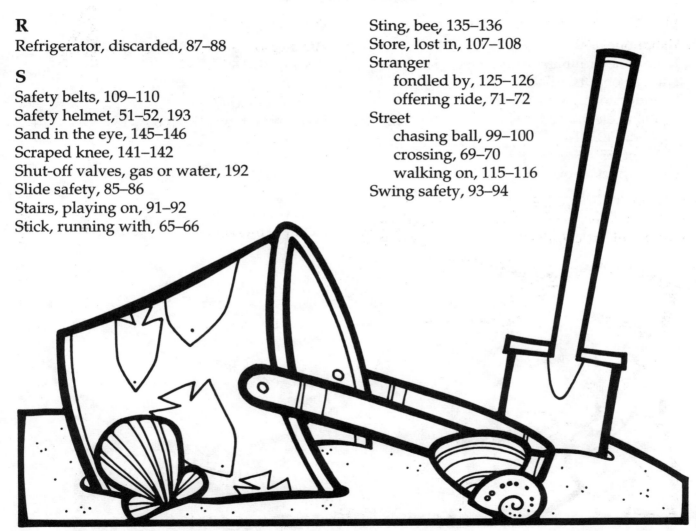

Index
(continued)

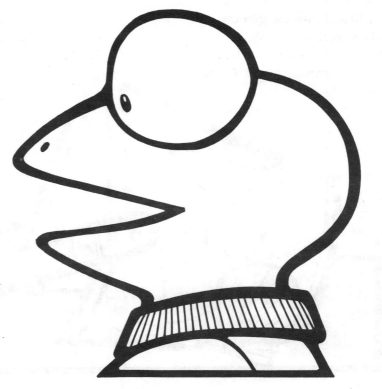

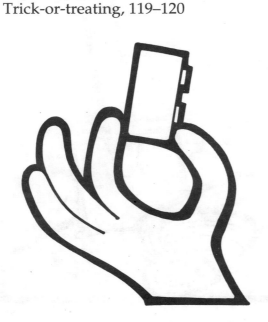